PRAISE FOR
AMERICAN DETOX

"Kerri Kelly has written us an intimate, honest, accountable, and thorough invitation into healing with *American Detox*. We won't heal unless we are willing to let go of colonizing the planet and our own bodies. We won't heal until we face ourselves. With vulnerable storytelling, grounded politics, and guided self-reflection, Kelly shows us a way to move past the capitalist myth of wellness into the possibility of true healing."

> —adrienne maree brown, writer-in-residence at the Emergent Strategy Ideation Institute whose work focuses on pleasure activism, emergent strategy, visionary fiction, and abolition

"We have built a culture of wellness from the master's tools of American capitalism, white supremacist delusion, and disconnection; and yet we continue to wonder why so many of us are deeply unwell. Late poet Audre Lorde told us that 'the master's tools will not dismantle the master's house.' *American Detox* carries on in this tradition, reminding us that we cannot purchase our way into well-being. It is built of the materials of interconnectedness and belonging, and without them we can't manifest the highest form of wellness which is humanity's wholeness."

> —SONYA RENEE TAYLOR, author of the *New York Times* best seller, *The Body Is Not an Apology*

"Kerri Kelly is radically committed to our well-being by teaching us how to 'be well'—within ourselves and with one another."

> —LAYLA F. SAAD, *New York Times* best-selling author of *Me and White Supremacy*

"Kerri Kelly has done her work. This book is a powerhouse. For anyone who cares deeply and yearns to live a meaningful life, one that yokes your most private moments with public actions and values, this book is a graceful and practical map. Full of research as well as intimate narrative, *American Detox* shows that how we do something is how we do everything."

—ASHLEY JUDD, American actress and political activist

"Kerri Kelly models deep solidarity in her being and breath. In the face of violence and terror, Kerri has grieved with me at the sites of massacre, joined her story to mine, and stood with me to hold up a vision of a world where we are all safe and free. Her debut book is a beautifully rendered reckoning with what ails this nation and the medicine we need to heal. *American Detox* is a blueprint for collective wellness, from an activist and healer who walks the walk with integrity, grace, and a revolutionary love."

—VALARIE KAUR, Sikh activist and best-selling author of
See No Stranger

"*American Detox* is the medicine this country needs right now. Urgent and unflinching, it exposes the structural and interpersonal practices that prevent us all from being well. Whether we're looking to change our systems or change ourselves, Kelly's words act, guide, and rally us toward the future we deserve."

—NICOLE CARDOZA, founder of Reclamation Ventures,
author, and magician

"This book offers the reframe that is needed in a culture desperately seeking wellness and perfection while being bankrupt of the remembrance of our inherent wholeness. Thank you, Kerri Kelly, for providing accessible tools to reclaim our well-being."

—TRACEE STANLEY, best-selling author of *Radiant Rest*

"Kerri, with her trademark dedication to fierce and honest self-examination, holds both herself and the culture of wellness accountable for the social dis-ease that continues to segregate health among its diverse citizenry. *American Detox* disrupts the myth of who gets to be well, exposes the constructs that benefit from people being ill, and provides insights into what needs to be done, individually and collectively, so that ALL beings have access to what they need in order to thrive."

—SEANE CORN, author of *Revolution of the Soul*

"For many years, Kerri Kelly has been on the front lines of and firmly planted at the intersection of social justice and well-being. *American Detox* is not only a wake-up call but a call to remember if some of us aren't well, none of us are well. This book shares a history of how individualism, competition, supremacy, and superiority have been embedded in the industry of wellness since its inception, and offers a way for us to detox from what no longer serves the collective while inviting us to come back to one another through practices of collective care. It is a must-read for the times in which we live and a guide for a pathway toward healing."

—MICHELLE JOHNSON, author of *Finding Refuge*

"Kerri is not afraid to ask the hard questions or face difficult truths! *American Detox* challenges us to examine and confront the systems of injustice that cut us off from our belonging to each other and from our wholeness of spirit. A brilliant call for the reimagining of what it means to be well in our world."

—TARA BRACH, author of *Trusting the Gold*

"As delicious as green juice is, it will not save us. Compassionate and critical inquiry into the systems that limit access to being well for so many in our world, now, that will. Is the way we do wellness well? In *American Detox* Kerri Kelly boldly asks us to examine that question in truth and light. She asks us to get curious and to look into personal and collective dark spaces in order to more clearly see how deeply unwell we are. This book is a valiant, brave, and timely compass and tool that we need right now as so many navigate the often wild, predatory, and ailing space of the so-called wellness industry."

—OCTAVIA RAHEEM, founder of Starshine & Clay, a meditation and yoga studio for Black women and women of color, and author of *Pause, Rest, Be*

"*American Detox* promotes well-being for all beings. In it, Kerri Kelly casts a vital, beautiful light into the dark corners of spirituality and wellness culture, helping to illuminate the true meaning of wellness and redefining 'self-help' to transform not just individual people—but as a call-to-action to improve the wellness of our communities and the world at large, too."

—SAH D'SIMONE, spiritual revolutionary and best-selling author of *5-Minute Daily Meditations*

THE MYTH OF
WELLNESS AND
HOW WE CAN
TRULY HEAL

AMERICAN DETOX

KERRI KELLY

Foreword by Rev. angel Kyodo williams

North Atlantic Books

Huichin, unceded Ohlone land
aka Berkeley, California

Published by
North Atlantic Books
Huichin, unceded Ohlone land
aka Berkeley, California

Cover design by Jess Morphew
Book design by Happenstance Type-O-Rama

Printed in the United States of America

American Detox: The Myth of Wellness and How We Can Truly Heal is sponsored and published by North Atlantic Books, an educational nonprofit based in the unceded Ohlone land Huichin (*aka* Berkeley, CA), that collaborates with partners to develop cross-cultural perspectives, nurture holistic views of art, science, the humanities, and healing, and seed personal and global transformation by publishing work on the relationship of body, spirit, and nature.

North Atlantic Books' publications are distributed to the US trade and internationally by Penguin Random House Publishers Services. For further information, visit our website at www.northatlanticbooks.com.

Library of Congress Cataloging-in-Publication Data

Names: Kelly, Kerri
Title: American detox : wellness in times of injustice and how we heal
   ourselves and the world / Kerri Kelly.
Description: Huichin, unceded Ohlone land aka Berkeley, California : North
   Atlantic Books, 2022. | Includes bibliographical references and index.
Identifiers: LCCN 2021057638 (print) | LCCN 2021057639 (ebook) | ISBN
   9781623177249 (trade paperback) | ISBN 9781623177256 (ebook)
Subjects: LCSH: Social change—United States. | Social action—United
   States. | Hope—United States.
Classification: LCC HN65 .K45 2022 (print) | LCC HN65 (ebook) | DDC
   303.40973—dc23/eng/20211201
LC record available at https://lccn.loc.gov/2021057638
LC ebook record available at https://lccn.loc.gov/2021057639

1 2 3 4 5 6 7 8 9 KPC 27 26 25 24 23 22

This book includes recycled material and material from well-managed forests. North Atlantic Books is committed to the protection of our environment. We print on recycled paper whenever possible and partner with printers who strive to use environmentally responsible practices.

For my mother,

*who taught me how to
be a strong feminist
without knowing it.*

This book is for you.

CONTENTS

FOREWORD

We were headed into the 2012 election, with Barack Obama running for his second term. I'd spent the last four years dismayed by how under-engaged the well-meaning white convert Buddhists that I'd come up around were. After the shock of a Black man being swept into the highest office in the land I let myself believe that some small corner had been turned. I certainly didn't think we were "post-racial," as people hilariously trotted out, but I did expect there to be some kind of meaningful engagement. I even wrote an essay, *Finally American*, as an ode to feeling a connection to that concept taken for granted by white people—being American—that had eluded me for all of my politically conscious life. I thought that having put themselves on the line to get him voted in, those same "good" white people would support him.

When it turned out that the white people I thought were "good" overwhelmingly weren't actually voting, I was simply not having it. Like any good spiritual activist, I needed to not just sit there, but do something.

I grew up Black and queer in New York, thumping, jumping, and blasting the beats of misogynist hip-hop while steering an organization that would help define the Third Wave of feminism. Contradictions, anyone? Eventually, I was called into formal Zen meditation practice, which offered me a way to transmute pain I'd held without having an answer for "why?" Through yoga, I found my way back into a body that had been the subject of secret violences and violation visited on me as a child by people that I loved and eventually learned had endured great violence themselves. In earth-based practices, my disconnect from the natural world began to dissolve.

These equipped me with an ability to be integrated and hold complexity, but also steadied my unwillingness to not name what was present. As I saw how the movements of my time were being consumed by the culture they were steeped in—urgency, aggression, and relentless competition—I joined with a loose network of other people committed to justice and grounded by spiritual practice who knew a transformation of the larger culture was called for. The inner-meets-outer of what we had been calling "this work" needed a name. I coined the phrase *Transformative Social Change* to speak to the idea that without inner change there can be no outer change and without collective change no change matters.

I was led to Kerri because we'd had the same epiphany: the so-called higher-level consciousness of the spiritual-not-religious-mystic-nondual-east-meets-west paradigm had spawned what is arguably one of the most disruptive industries to run counter to the aggressive American Marlboro-meets-Madmen, hyper-masculine, hyper-individualistic narrative: wellness.

The wellness world had all the right principles—nonviolence, compassion, ecological consciousness, interdependence. Why wouldn't they have the "right" politics? We both saw enormous potential that could be unleashed for good. We just needed to get them off their om-ing, so-peaceful-I-can't-be-bothered asses and to the polls. So in 2012 that's what we set out to do.

I like to say that Kerri Kelly and I share an unlikely *twinship*. There we were, New Yorkers in California and in no time at all, it was revealed that not only were we from the place where people actually say what they mean, but also we both have fireman fathers nicknamed "Butch." From the beginning, we shared an awareness of how our various "identities" intersected and shaped us. It wasn't just an obligatory politeness. We were implicitly saying, "you need to know this about me," and embedded within that, the many possible lines of convergence and divergence. Class was named. Race was explicit. The demands, points of access, and limitations of our respective locations were laid bare. We weren't just telling each other where we were from, we were telling each other where we were *from*.

The whole "we'll just get them to vote" project didn't turn out well. Two conventions and a month of exhaustion later, we realized that the problem wasn't generic apathy: it was whiteness.

This is where *American Detox* comes in.

American Detox is the kind of book that is going to catch some flack. You can't challenge the status quo and expect that it won't ruffle feathers. If Kerri had written a book that simply extended the caboose of the culture of vitriol, finger-pointing, shaming, and canceling that we now desperately cling to to avoid having that finger pointed our way, lots of us could happily hop on the bandwagon and parade above the avenue on our high and mighty, smart-ass, progressive hovercrafts, sailing over the ever-growing "basket of deplorables." All the people we don't agree with or like, that don't have the right politics, aren't woke enough, don't keep up with the latest lingo, or just can't afford to get on . . . well, they will just burn as we sail above it all.

But *American Detox* doesn't stop at ruffling feathers, it swipes-left the platforms that we stand on and pontificate from. It's an ocean of truth-telling that swallows up all the ways we hide from treading into the deep waters of "who am I *really* when so much of what I believed myself to be has been shaped by a culture that never wanted me to see beyond the veil?"

Little by little, the straight look into the face of falsehoods we were weaned on plunges daggers into the chinks in the armor of domination-thinking that keeps some of us cocooned in a narcotic sense of safety.

No doubt some Black and brown folks may take umbrage at a white woman talking about race, 'cause—you know—the system of capitalism favors and rewards white women and white people generally, even when they are saying the things we couldn't say without getting hurt or killed. It's a fair critique and an understandable place of pain for many of us. I say that from firsthand experience of having my first book, a primer on Zen Buddhism, dismissed by some as a "Black book," while white self-proclaimed Buddhist women could write about their experience and that didn't make it a "white book."

And yet...us Black and brown folks have spent a long, long time telling white folks to "go get your people." We won't change the system by who we hold back but by supporting those we trust and *can get through the gates* to go forth and throw wrenches in the gears of the system until they will cease to turn. Kerri walks with a pocket full of wrenches.

The beauty and the blessing is that in *American Detox*, Kerri doesn't wave a smug flag from atop a mountain of knowing. She walks the journey of asking the questions with us every step of the way. Not showing us "how it's done," but pointing at resources and practices we might use to begin to undo it—if we choose to. *American Detox* is presented like good medicine: a bitter pill to swallow, but confident in the healing that comes about when a living system is relieved of the toxicity that overwhelms it. There's an abiding trust that whoever we are, when we strip the layers away, let the toxic beliefs and ways of thinking and being be confronted and allowed to flow through and out of our systems, we are worthy of returning to a basic wholeness.

Not getting somewhere. Returning.

There's no promise to become super, better, uber, extra, more anything, but you. And not alone. Together. As a collective member of humanity. As Taj James reminds us,

To the last breath, we are not afraid. Because we know who we are, and we know we are a continuation of those who came before us, and we know those who come after us will be a continuation of us, and there is nothing to fear.

—*Rev. angel Kyodo williams, writer, activist, ordained Zen priest, and author of* Radical Dharma

Waking Up

> For a seed to achieve its greatest expression, it must come completely undone. The shell cracks, its insides come out and everything changes. To someone who doesn't understand growth, it would look like complete destruction.
>
> CYNTHIA OCCELLI

If you have come for a quick fix, I'm afraid you've come to the wrong place. This book will not offer some magic pill, life hack, or wellness protocol for living longer or looking younger. Rather this is about the messy and vulnerable work of transformative change. The kind of change that demands the whole truth and nothing but the truth. The kind of change that becomes impossible to avoid when the world falls apart.

That moment for me was 9/11. I lost my stepfather, my city, and my entire sense of safety and normal. The life that I'd been living and the person that I'd been before 9/11 were destroyed. And I was left to pick up the pieces and make sense of my new reality. 9/11/2001

There is no handbook for how to survive the unimaginable. There is only what you have learned and what you are capable of. At the time, I had an all-American, middle-class upbringing at my back and a yoga and meditation practice to keep me sane. It was the latter that saved my ass.

The wellness world had all the answers to my questions. It offered relief from the grief and pain. It promised to make me thinner and more productive. It told me to look on the bright side of my really shitty situation. And before long, I was hooked, aggressively seeking self-help, self-discovery, self-perfection, self-everything. I would hit my mat, stalk organic food, and seek exotic retreats like my life depended on it.

But when I stepped outside of the bliss and safety of my mat, I was confronted with a very different reality. The world outside of my wellness bubble was different. Really different. Everyday families struggling to survive, children going to school hungry, guns ripping apart entire communities, families losing their homes to the mortgage crisis, people denied human rights and dignity because of the color of their skin, their religion, their sexual orientation. Nonstop policing, incarcerating, deporting, bombing.

I began to grapple with why I got to be well when others didn't. How well-being had somehow become a privilege afforded to people with access and time and money. People like me. Which drove me to the inquiry explored in this book—whether a culture of wellness that refuses to consider the well-being of all is actually making things worse for everyone.

The Myth of Wellness

Wellness—the industry that grew out of self-help and fitness classes and has exploded into everything from yoga to crystals to juice cleanses—promises to make you better, stronger, healthier, and whole. It meets an ever-increasing demand among many Americans to "feel good" and find meaning in a cruel and confusing world. And it's no wonder. In the face of rising health threats, extreme inequality, endless wars, and our own possible extinction, it makes sense that we would seek relief.

But wellness isn't just the yearning to be well. It is extreme materialism masquerading as spiritual practice to make us feel good while emptying our wallets. It is the commoditization of political ideas like "self-care" and "empowerment" as something that you can buy. And it is a $4.5 trillion global industry that is servicing the millions of people like me who are desperate to be well.[1]

But while wellness soars, so does inequality.

2

Inequality has been the purpose of the so-called American Dream for as long as we've had one. Colonization, slavery, and capitalism have resulted in a legacy of unequal conditions that runs as deep as well water. A recent study found the US to be the wealthiest among developed nations—and the most unequal.[2] While certain populations are making choices about organic and GMO-free food, the rest of the country is trying to figure out how to feed their families *and* pay their bills.

The truth is that we—the big *we*—are not well. Not by a long shot.

I call it the **well-being gap**: the unequal conditions that determine who gets to be well and who doesn't.[3] It is a disparity driven not by personal choice but by proximity to power and privilege. And it goes way beyond the affordability or accessibility of wellness products and services. Wherever there is a prevalence of poverty and unemployment, a lack of access to housing and healthcare, people are struggling to survive much less be well. But a well-being gap that leaves many people behind ultimately hurts all of us. It destabilizes our economy, it causes stress that makes us sick, it fuels higher rates of crime and violence, it holds back our children, and it creates an ever deeper divide among neighbors and neighborhoods.

But that's not the only thing. Everywhere we turn, culture gaslights us with the message that "we're not good enough." It says, "Buy this and you will be happy," "Do this and you will feel beautiful," "Eat this and you will be healthy," "Read this and you will be enlightened." It is a storyline sponsored by a system that profits from our sickness.

The wellness industry sells us isolation and escapism. It dangles the false promise of perfection and purity. And we are just left more alone, more dissatisfied, and more isolated than ever. Fixating on self-help, self-seeking, self-everything keeps us fending for ourselves, neglecting the suffering of our friends and neighbors, and denying our humanity.

Wellness is not making us well. It's making us worse. While wellness promises enlightenment, the circumstances of our lived reality tell a different story. The many crises we are facing are exponential—from infectious disease to racial injustice, to extreme income inequality, to accelerating climate change. And while wellness exploits our fears and vulnerabilities, it does nothing to address the systems that got us here in the first place. It blames us for our struggles but refuses to acknowledge what's at the root of our suffering.

To make things worse, most of today's wellness industry draws on a lineage of mind-body practices, largely from South Asian and Indigenous cultures, that are often a part of spiritual traditions that employ a holistic and collectivist approach to well-being. Yet these practices have been divorced from their original contexts, distorted, and commodified to accommodate racist capitalist culture. In this book I do my best to uncover these truths and how the wellness industry itself has become a weapon of dominant systems to maintain the status quo and distract people from reality. Despite our desperate pursuit, wellness is not making us well. Well-being is a human right, not a privilege. And my well-being is not isolated or separate from yours. That means that true wellness demands that we confront everything that is in the way of our collective well-being.*

No amount of green juice or hybrid cars is going to save the planet. Meditation is not going to undo systemic racism. Ecotourism is not going to solve inequality. But wellness sells us the idea that we can buy our way to well-being. I bought into that myth. I traded in my corporate ambition for wellness purity and realized that it was just more of the same: a constant cycle that keeps us stuck in the status quo and starving for more. And while it is easy to turn away and stay in our gated communities of wellness, we must turn toward the hard-to-look-at truth of our people and planet and demand more of ourselves and one another.

Toxic Culture

The myth of wellness is a symptom of a toxic culture steeped in separation, scarcity, and supremacy. It is the legacy of colonization, slavery, and exploitation that has shaped America's dominant story and collective consciousness. Dominant culture tells us not to look, not to acknowledge the horrors that are all around us. It teaches us to rationalize inequality and

---

* Well-being and wellness are not the same. I define *well-being* as the state of being well or feeling whole, whereas *wellness* is the active pursuit of well-being.

justify harm. It encourages us to fend for ourselves at the expense of others. It overwhelms us with information and confuses us with lies. It decides who is "normal" and worthy of well-being. And it does whatever is necessary to remain in control and in power. Whether we like it or not, all of us are situated in this culture and socialized to play our assigned roles to keep the system in place.

Socialization is the process of inducting an individual into the social world. It is how we learn the norms, values, standards, and expectations of us within a group or whole society. It is not inherently bad. Socialization is how resilience gets passed down from generation to generation. But it is also how we have inherited and internalized racism and other systems of oppression over hundreds of years. In this context, socialization becomes a systematic training of "how to be" in the dynamic systems of oppression. Powerful forces, including institutions, mass media, and technology, operate to influence and enforce our participation in the system. Bobbie Harro, sociologist and author of *The Cycle of Socialization*, says that this cycle "'teaches' us how to play our assigned roles in oppression, and how to revere the existing systems that shape our thinking, leading us to blame uncontrollable forces, other people, or ourselves for the existence of oppression."[4] This process, like culture itself, is consistent, circular, self-perpetuating, and often invisible in the way that it lands on us and in us.

Culture operates like water. It is slippery and fluid, often shape-shifting into whatever keeps the system in place. We are molded and manipulated by its force. All of us swim in this water whether we like it or not. It is impossible to avoid, permeating every tissue and cell in our bodies. Socialization is how we learn to "swim" in this water—it teaches stereotypes, fosters comparison, normalizes oppression, and demands obedience. This operating system is always functioning in the background, informing our relationships, institutions, and culture. When the water is toxic, we become immersed in ideas of separation, scarcity, and supremacy that shape our bodies and minds and work against our personal and collective well-being. Ultimately, it becomes the frame through which we see and respond to the world.

American Detox is a radical reckoning with the realization that there can be no well-being of *me* without a well-being of *we*. It tells the truth about where we are as a country, how we got here, and what it's gonna take to transform ourselves from the inside out. It challenges ideas of scarcity and self-preservation and inspires us to imagine better and to go from futility to possibility, from individualism to mutual responsibility, from treating symptoms to transforming systems, from winning at all costs to working across difference, from policies of fear to revolutionary love, and from a well-being of me to a well-being of we.

Showing Up for the Work

This is not some prophetic rant by a self-proclaimed thought leader. Quite the opposite. Like so many of us, I was brought up to follow the rules and fall in line. Trained to check off the boxes, climb the ladder, and live the "American Dream." I bought into that dream the same way I bought into the myth of wellness—through the idea that I was not already whole, enough, healthy, and strong. I had been molded and shaped into the consummate "good girl," loved for my conformity and rewarded for my obedience. Between the guilt of my Catholic upbringing, the aspiration of my family, the competition of my schooling, and the ambition of corporate America, I was indoctrinated into a culture that had me hustling to be perfect. Wellness was just more of the same.

But my obsession with wellness wasn't making me well. Not because of my yearning to be whole, but because of my belief that I could buy my way into it, that I could escape the truth of who we are and how we got here. Wellness is just one more system that has been colonized by ideologies of individualism, white supremacy, ableism, and capitalism. And until we wake up to it—until we begin to interrogate the systems that thrive off convincing us that we are not good enough; that shame the aging process and deny the certainty of dying; that sell enlightenment and peace of mind under the cloak of capitalism; that preach of "oneness" while dividing, excluding, and exploiting; and that idolize the self at the expense of the whole—we will remain imprisoned by its hand.

Questions, not answers, brought me to this book. I wanted to know how we got here and what it's going to take to really heal. And I wanted to own my part, to share how I am both implicated and impacted, both a part of the problem and a part of the solution. You will find that I am not afraid to share the messy details of my becoming. I am not afraid to be wrong and acknowledge my willful ignorance as a growing person. I'm not afraid to name the systems of oppression, like white supremacy, patriarchy, and ableism, that have molded me into the very soldier that I am at war with. I am not afraid to be a traitor to my kind, to bite the hand that feeds me, so long as the truth is set free. I'm willing to take the risk of exposing myself because I believe that the stakes are too high for us to remain stuck and scared.

For the last two decades, I have worked at the intersection of well-being and justice—navigating the relationship between inner change and outer change, between the individual and the collective, between the personal and political, between me and we. In all these places, I have tried to play my part—to listen, tell the truth, expose harm, demand integrity, and explore the unimaginable, often messy experiences of transformation. I have learned that there is no right or wrong, no binary answers to complex, intersectional questions. The dissonance and discomfort that have emerged from this practice have been my greatest teacher, encouraging me to question everything, to be relentless in pursuit of the truth, to examine where I am out of integrity, and to do my part in confronting the beast within myself and all around me.

Along the way, I've had the privilege of learning with community organizers, social activists, policy makers, and spiritual leaders in a shared exploration of the relationship between inner work and outer change. I've sat at the table with company executives who are navigating social impact and the art of doing good while not doing harm. I've organized alongside fast-food workers, Black women, dreamers, and pro-choice feminists who all share an understanding that our liberation and well-being are bound. I've marched, boycotted, testified, lobbied, and gotten arrested. I've tried, failed, fucked up, and started over. And all of it has taught me that wellness isn't what we *do* on the mat or the cushion, it's who we *be* in the world. It's how we live into our relationship to each other and to all living things. And it's how we find our way home—how we do whatever is necessary to repair what has been broken, how we reckon with whatever is in the way of our collective well-being—and return to living in ecological balance and harmony.

We were born into a toxic world. There is no retreat, no ashram or homestead, that is immune to the culture of separation, scarcity, and supremacy that we are all a part of. For us to be truly well, we need to detoxify ourselves from the ideologies that have shaped our reality—from a white supremacy that says some lives are more valuable than others; from a capitalism that values productivity and profits over people; and from an individualism that keeps us separate and denies our interconnectedness.

This Moment

Which brings me to this moment—where in the face of a world-altering pandemic, a deteriorating democracy, and an increasingly undeniable changing-climate crisis, there is a huge push to get back to "normal." But what is the normal we are getting back to? An America built on stolen land? An America financed by enslavement? An America that has put progress and profit over people and planet? Normal is a lie that ignores and avoids the unbearable past we come from and the unjust present we inhabit. And given the rate of acceleration, it is going to cost us our future.

Since 9/11 alone, we've seen an erosion of private and civil liberties, the expansion of the surveillance state, a so-called war on terror that has cost more than a million lives, an increase in deportation, a rise in white nationalism, and an ever more unequal America. The lie of a "post-racial" United States that was popularized after the election of Barack Obama was painfully exposed under Donald Trump. Trump's America was not new but a brutal reminder of the story we have refused to tell—the story about who we really are and how we really got here. The country of life, liberty, and the pursuit of happiness is also a country of stealing land, exploiting bodies, and upholding supremacy.

And yet, as America teeters on the brink of destruction, the wellness industry has swelled to an all-time high, growing exponentially in the last twenty years and servicing a massive movement of self-care, mindfulness,

and conscious consumption in the US today. It is a paradox of epic proportions. The myth of well-being isn't making us better. And until we reckon
with the truth of how we got here, detoxify ourselves from the culture of
separation, and repair our relationship to one another, we won't ever realize the aspiration of the American project. *American Detox* is not a rejection
of America but a longing for what could be. Some will read this book and
call me unpatriotic for my analysis and criticism. But I believe nothing is
more patriotic than challenging ourselves to become the country we are
capable of—which is only possible when all of us can participate fully.

American Detox is not a rejection of wellness but a reclaiming of it. Because
we can't talk about wellness until we talk about the violence of white supremacy. We can't talk about wellness until we talk about the myth of normalcy.
We can't talk about wellness until we talk about the addiction to perfectionism. We can't talk about wellness until we talk about the exploitation of labor
and the degradation of our planet. We can't talk about wellness until we talk
about the very real well-being gap that determines who gets to be well and
who doesn't. In the pages that follow, I attempt to hold this tension between
who we are and who we are striving to become. To acknowledge complicity
as a starting point for healing. To name the truth of our history, the reality of
culture and socialization, the cost of privilege and oppression, while simultaneously creating space for radical practice and possibility. It is a practice of
"both/and"—an invitation to hold the paradox of our existence in modern
times and navigate our way through with grace and resilience.

We are a nation at a crossroads: Will we continue to devolve into white
supremacist extremism, toxic individualism, and economic extraction and
to accelerate toward our extinction? Or will we do what is necessary to heal
our wounds, repair our relationships, and build the more beautiful country
that we all deserve? How we show up in this moment will determine who
we are as a community and as a nation.

Reimagining Well-Being

This book is for people like me who are waking up to insidious systems of
domination and reckoning with their place in it. But it is also for anyone

who is yearning to be healed, to be whole, to be well. I wrote it for the inse-cure little girl I once was, who thought she had to be good and perfect to be loved. I wrote it for the overachiever inside of me who was taught to always strive for more because I'm never enough. It is for the corporate climber, the wellness enthusiast, the ambitious activist, the white savior, and the many other versions of me who learned the hard way that there is no true freedom or well-being in a culture of separation, scarcity, and supremacy. This book is for the person I was when I didn't know, the person I am today who is still trying to figure it out, and the person I am becoming that is a big, messy work in progress.

Of course, this book was written from my *personal* location—my lived experience in the US and all that I have inherited from its history. It also comes from my *social* location—where and how I am situated in relationship to sys-tems of power and privilege. Being a white, cisgender, straight, nondisabled citizen in America affords me an array of advantages I didn't earn, which not only implicates me in systems of oppression but shapes my perspective. The learning and wisdom I put forth in this book are only possible because of the legacy of resistance by Black people, Indigenous folks, other people of color, disability justice organizers, and LGBTQIA activists. The American project wouldn't be what it is today if those who were excluded from its orig-inal vision didn't fight for the realization of "life, liberty, and the pursuit of happiness" for all. This book is a humble attempt to honor their legacy and do my part in helping build a just world where everyone can thrive.

It is in the spirit of this commitment that led me to the inquiry I present in this book: How do we face the truth of who we are and how we got here? How do we navigate the toxicity of this moment, and where do we go from here? How do we show up as citizens of humanity for the well-being of the whole?

You won't find step-by-step instructions or one-size-fits-all solutions for how to be well and make change. Rather, I invite you, the reader, to join me on a journey of personal reckoning, radical truth-telling, and shared prac-tice that brings forth a culture of collective well-being, a new-old paradigm that is **interdependent**, **radical**, and **resilient**. Interdependent in how it affirms that we are not separate from one another and from the planet. Radical in how it demands that we go to the root and reclaim the whole story of who we are and how we got here. And resilient in how we stay engaged and diligent, even when it gets hard.

This book follows my own humble story from 9/11 to now and how I have had to grapple with what it means to be well in a fucked-up world. It was not some blossoming into blissfulness but rather a tale of coming undone, of looking at my own narcissism, racism, and discrimination and taking responsibility for my part in this mess. I come to this work having lived it, having reckoned with my own hypocrisy and humanness, and believing that we can do better. My stories are in service to the process of transformation and the detoxification and discovery that are necessary for true well-being to emerge.

Each chapter exposes a cultural myth that has kept me—and so many people in my life—stuck. It invites a critical lens on wellness culture and how it manifests in perfectionism, isolation, individualism, white supremacy, and apathy. In an effort to understand how we got here, I do my best to tell the truth about history, to expose the events that steered our course, to name the systems that hold us back, and to invite inquiry into how our bodies and minds are infected by the toxic systems and culture and what it is costing us. At the end of each chapter, I grapple with recovery: what it looks like to detox and untangle our bodies and minds from these harmful ideologies and how to create liberatory conditions where everyone can thrive. It is not a prescription or magic pill but an everyday practice of waking up, getting free, and showing up for the well-being of the whole. It affirms that the well-being so many of us are relentlessly seeking can only be realized together through collective care and action. And in the book's final chapter, with the help of movement leaders on the front lines of love and justice, we will reimagine the future of well-being that we all deserve.

American Detox is an invitation to go on a journey that is both critical and compassionate. Along the way, we will consider how we got here, our past wounds—personal and collective—and how we have been shaped by them. We will contemplate power and enoughness and our role in changing the course for our people and planet. We will learn how to love again—a radical and revolutionary love that heals and repairs our social fabric. We will find each other through solidarity and speaking truth to power. We will imagine beyond the status quo, dreaming up new systems that take care of everyone. We will emerge into our purposeful role as engaged citizens for humanity.

This book is written for all of us, all of us who are willing to ask hard questions about who we are and who we are to one another, and what's possible when we liberate ourselves from the toxicity of oppressive systems and show up for the well-being of everyone. I hope it stirs you up. I hope it excavates old and stubborn ground, so that it can be composted into new and fertile soil. I hope it makes you curious about what you don't know and accepting of what you can't understand. I hope it makes you outraged and also gives you hope. I hope it inspires you to show up and do something different. And I hope it calls you to reimagine a future of well-being that works for all of us, not just some of us.

CHAPTER 1

Ground Zero

> Your pain is the breaking of the shell that encloses your understanding.
>
> KHALIL GIBRAN

Before

Early morning was always my favorite time in New York. An overture before the curtain goes up, when the city starts buzzing with potential. I felt a real part of the city during this time, like a stagehand privy to the behind-the-scenes show. I loved waking up to the sounds of delivery trucks and traffic, to store owners opening their doors, to coffee brewing and eggs frying in bodegas.

As I blazed down Madison Avenue, I would join the stream of commuters as they flowed toward their workplaces. New Yorkers know how to move—weaving between blocks and buildings, dodging cars, and racing traffic lights. It is deliberate. There is no idle in Manhattan, a city as driven as its inhabitants. We were a mighty river of people flowing between concrete banks toward purpose and productivity.

This particular day in September was no exception. But it was even more brilliant than usual—one of those stubborn summer days pushing up against fall with all of its strength. I noticed how the sun bounced off the buildings, creating a prism effect that lit up the street and made shadows dance across the pavement. I appreciated this beauty, but I was not stalled by it. After all, productivity was our currency here; it's what defined us, how we proved our existence and our worth. And I was all in.

First to the office, I settled into a desk nestled among others just like it. There was no privacy, just enough office dividers to optimize isolation and output. Straight off of a vacation, I felt refreshed and determined to take advantage of this surge of energy. I was early in my career in media/advertising and driven. I knew this ladder and I was climbing it fast and furiously. A relentless overachiever since childhood, I was made for corporate America and I planned on ruling it.

I didn't even notice as people trickled in. It wasn't until someone knocked on my door that I lifted my head out of my zone.

"Have you heard?"

"What?" I responded, slightly annoyed at the disruption.

"A plane hit the World Trade Center."

"Holy shit. What happened?"

"I don't know."

I turned the radio on, put my head down, and got back to work. A few minutes later, I heard screaming and chaos coming from the radio. A second plane had hit the second tower. This was no accident.

I called my mom.

"Do you see what's happening?"

"Yeah," she said. "I haven't talked to Joe yet."

"What do you mean? Isn't he home?"

"Kerri, he's working."

I hung up the phone and everything slowed down. Joe was my stepdad and a lieutenant at Ladder 15 in South Street Seaport. I pictured the firehouse tucked in the shadow of the towers a few short blocks away. I imagined him there giving orders and taking care of his men. He was always there when you needed him. It was exactly how he'd showed up for my mom and me twenty years earlier. The hairs stuck up on the back of my neck. And even as my thoughts started to race, there were places I wouldn't let my mind go. Everything was going to be fine. I just needed to keep it together.

By this time people were starting to huddle in the office and trade information. There was no more talk of work. We were being attacked. New York. The city of the invincible, attacked.

"My brother works down there."

"My wife said she saw papers all over the ground in Battery Park."

"I just talked to my cousin who said people are jumping from the buildings."

Information moves at the speed of light in New York. From coworker to cousin to deli owner to doorman, it's always an intricate human web of information and gossip. But today information was like oxygen—desperately needed and life-giving.

We gathered in my director's office around a TV. All of us, crammed in, watching buildings burn and sharing this strange and horrifying experience as it played out before our very eyes. There was a silence beneath the words.

Then, the unimaginable happened. At first we couldn't believe our eyes. The tower didn't fall like one would imagine. It didn't lean or tip on its side or break off. It just . . . fell . . . into itself. It took me a minute to realize what I was witnessing. People were yelling, I think. I can't be sure. The sound was sucked out of the room, and something broke inside of me. It was like I was witnessing myself split into two. One part of me was clinging to an almost irrational hope. Joe was probably not in the building. He was a lieutenant now. He would hang back and give orders from mission control.

But there was this other part of me—a deeper part of me—that had this felt sense. He was there. Of course he was. He'd do the thing he'd always done. He would run directly into that building and step into the fire.

Later we would recover the radio transmissions detailing his final moments in the tower. He was last heard calling out to his men at 9:57 a.m., just two minutes before the second tower came down. He was trapped in a stairwell on the floor of impact, and the walls were caving in. His final words: "I'll be right to you."

I don't need to tell you the rest of the story. It all just ends there, in that moment, at 9:59 a.m. on September 11, 2001. Buried in the rubble of those buildings is my former life. I can never go back. None of us can. I was forever changed.

When Things Fall Apart

The immediate aftermath of 9/11 was a thing to behold. Two of the tallest buildings in the world, and a symbol of prosperity and power, reduced to rubble. A toxic cloud of pulverized architecture and debris cloaked Manhattan. The smell of smoke, burning debris, and death hung in the air, and people streamed in all directions. They were covered in dust, clinging to one other. First responders frantically clawed the pile for survivors, for bodies, for hope.

What New Yorkers witnessed that day defied our imagination. It was as if we were transported to another time and place entirely. All remnants of "before" destroyed. This was the new reality, piled upon the old reality that lay buried deep beneath the surface. One could only imagine what else was down there, old histories and truths never to be recovered. The pile seemed insurmountable, and we, the survivors, were stripped bare, razed to the bone, defenseless.

In the immediate aftermath, questions were the only thing we had: What will happen next? What should we do? Who's right? Who's wrong? Who's to blame? We waded in a never-ending sea of uncertainty. And yet that moment was also a great revealer. Everything that had been hidden in the shadows, buried beneath the surface, came into view. We Americans were not invincible, not untouchable, no different from those who suffer around the globe. We were defenseless. We were human. And we were exposed.

After 9/11 my sense of meaning and belonging broke down. I was left with a world that no longer made sense. The life that I had built according to the all-American blueprint—the good job in Corporate America, the apartment on the Upper East Side, the fancy vacations and nice things, the skinny and fit body—all of a sudden felt ... wrong. I didn't know how to get up in the morning any more, much less be well.

As I moved from "he is missing" to "he is gone," from "we must find his body" to "we must find who is responsible," it wasn't anything I was prepared for. My family, my life, was broken in pieces and scattered across lower Manhattan. And I knew we would never be the same again. There was no instruction manual for how to survive that moment. But beneath the chaos and rubble, there was truth. Not the kind that was taught to me in school or church, but the real kind. The kind that can only come from within. A story that emerged from the cracks like a desperate gasp of air. It was as if the veil had been lifted and, for a brief moment, those of us who had lived in the shadow of the towers saw the truth about humanity, a humanity that is vulnerable and defenseless. And we saw each other and the preciousness of human life in this shared experience. A people inextricably tied in living and dying, in pain and suffering.

But as fast as those towers fell down, our walls flew up—shields of fear and hatred, distrust and division.

Shock and Awe

First there was shock and awe. "Shock and awe" was the term used by then President Bush to describe the US military campaign against Iraq in 2003, but it also adequately described our state of mind as a country on 9/11. Awe was the breath held, the mind suspended in shock, the rift in ordinary time. What happened that day was beyond our wildest imagination.

Next came desperation. An attempt to do anything to salvage what remained, to alleviate the despair, to save ourselves. Families of survivors plastered missing persons posters all over New York. First responders flooded down to Ground Zero from all corners of the globe. People gave blood, gave casseroles, gave kindness. Doing something, anything, gave us momentary respite from the pain, hope (however fleeting) that we would not be destroyed by this. Our first instinct was to reach out and help. There were even glimpses of joy amid the horror. In between the grief and uncertainty, I remember sweet moments of fellowship and generosity that I hadn't experienced before. For a brief time, we became the best version of ourselves. 9/11 gave us meaning—a feeling that there was something left of community, that there might be a purpose to all this destruction.

And then there was fear. Here's how fear works: something happens that scares you—a loud sound, a creepy crawler, a threatening stranger— and then the body prepares to protect itself. But when fear isn't realized or resolved, it gets imprinted in the body and normalized, shaping our beliefs and behaviors, and even our bodies. And with overexposure to triggering images in culture and media, we become predisposed to fear. Fear plays tricks with our minds, altering our perception of reality. It impacts our bodies, short-circuiting our rational response pathways, creating levels of stress, and manifesting as disease and dis-ease. We learn to live with our fear—even collude with it. To cope, we avoid, we numb, we get busy, we seek to control everything. Before we know it, fear becomes how we move in the world.

Fear is a powerful motivator. In evolutionary terms, fear is necessary to survive. But it also drives a dangerous us-vs.-them narrative that underlies some of the most horrific events of American history and everyday realities of American life. When we are afraid, we pull away from each other and give in to a culture of suspicion and distrust. Fear makes us strangers. And nearly two decades after 9/11, it is not the actual threat but the story of the threat that keeps our fear alive. In a 2020 Pew survey, Americans still ranked "defending the nation from terrorist attacks" as a top priority for the president and Congress,[1] even though jihadist terrorists have only killed about six people each year in the United States since 9/11—far more have been killed by hate crimes and homegrown extremists.[2] And yet, many in this country still remain afraid and have bought into false narratives of Arab, Muslim, and violent immigrant "others" that keep people tethered to a politics of fear, obedient to a militarized state, and beholden to authoritarian leaders.[*]

---

[*] To learn more about the aftermath of 9/11 from the perspective of Muslim, Sikh, and Arab people, read Deepa Kumar's *Islamophobia and the Politics of Empire*.

The dissonance between a real threat and irrational fear is important. Irrational fear is harder to eradicate and easily manipulated. The irony is that the fear, more than the terrorism, is what has done the most damage to this nation. Americans' desperate efforts to protect ourselves have increased our suffering and made us divided and distrustful. Fear has fueled policies of insecurity and inequality and enabled the dismantling of much-needed public services. It justified an enormous investment in the creation of the Department of Homeland Security and Immigration and Customs Enforcement—institutions fundamentally premised on compromising human rights and civil liberties in the name of mass surveillance, state violence, racist policing, incarceration, and deportation.* And it has conditioned us for war—a predisposition to conflict and conquest that goes back to the beginning of the American story and has enabled a military-industrial complex whose budget exceeds that of the next seven countries in military spending combined.

But at the end of the day, our fear doesn't make us safe. It only ends up serving the many industries and people that benefit from it. In her book *The Shock Doctrine* Naomi Klein describes the phenomenon of "disaster capitalism"—how institutions and corporations exploit the public's vulnerability and disorientation following a collective shock or trauma (e.g., wars, terrorist attacks, natural disasters, market crashes) to centralize control and push through pro-corporate, profit-driven initiatives.[3] Trump's "shock doctrine" took it a step further by manufacturing an "invasion" on our borders and using that to fuel anti-immigrant white populism, justify the travel ban against select Muslim-majority countries, build a wall, and separate children from their families. It is the worst kind of opportunism, exploiting the suffering of our most vulnerable moments for financial and political gain. This is modern-day America—a post-9/11 apocalypse fueling policies of fear and pulling us further apart from one another and from reality itself.

But this sort of deception is not new. It is woven into the fabric of our origin. The promise of American freedom for white European immigrants was only made possible on the backs of Indigenous Peoples and enslaved

---

* For more on the racist roots of the surveillance state, read *Dark Matters: On the Surveillance of Blackness* by Simone Browne.

Africans. The American Dream that emerged—the idea that equality and opportunity are available to any and all Americans—was more like an American lie. I bought into that lie. I was brainwashed to trust history books and idolize American icons of success and fame. I was groomed to strive— rewarded for getting good grades, being a tough competitor, and winning at all costs. Before I knew it, I was on an express train to some predetermined destination measured in achievement, money, and material goods. And for whatever reason, I never questioned it. I was trained to chase a dream that was never meant for me.

America was built on a false promise. All men were never "created equal" in the eyes of the founding fathers. The rights to life, liberty, and the pursuit of happiness certainly did not equally apply to Indigenous Peoples, enslaved people, women, and many others who did not fit into the founders' idea of the American ideal. This is the fault line in the foundation upon which the idea of America was built. It can no longer be ignored. It's why freedom has been so fraught over the last 400 years. To understand why we are here requires understanding how we got here and where we came from. The American experiment is yet to be realized, and to realize it, we must go back to the beginning.

Stolen Land

New York City is not just a place, it's an identity—a way of being in the world that is derived from hard work and tough love. Fast, boisterous, crowded, and adaptable, the City is a marvel, especially to those like me who get to call it home. New York, New York—the city of dreams—was built by immigrants. My ancestors were among them—Italian carpenters, Irish truck drivers, Jewish factory workers—all hustling to make it in America. I wore New York like a badge of honor—proof of my strength and resilience and all that I inherited from those who came before me. But despite our sweat and tears, New York never really belonged to us.

Before Ground Zero, before New York, before New Amsterdam, there was Lenapehoking. The land now known as Manhattan (as well as Westchester, Long Island, New Jersey, eastern Pennsylvania, and parts of Delaware) was stewarded by the Lenape people for 3,000 years before Europeans arrived. They were people who always understood that we are the land and the land is us. But explorers brought with them a different relationship with the land, one of domination and ownership. The first "land claim" came from Henry Hudson, representing the Dutch East India Company, who entered New York Bay on none other than September 11, 1609.[4]

For thousands of years before Columbus got lost at sea and accidentally found himself on the shores of a "new" world, generations of Indigenous Peoples lived and thrived on these lands. Of course, this is not the story I and many others learned in school. It was not a friendly Thanksgiving but a violent takeover with ideological roots that can be traced as far back as the fourth century, when Saint Augustine declared that war and killing are justified if they are in service to God.[5] A thousand years later, this Doctrine of Discovery would unleash a culture of domination and acquisition that became the bedrock upon which America was built. What followed was the legal and systemic dispossession and oppression of entire peoples, through broken treaties, forced relocations, outlawing Indigenous cultural and spiritual practices, hunting Indigenous food sources such as the buffalo to extinction, forced separation and Anglicization of children through the residential school system, and more. Colonizers are estimated to have killed tens of millions of people in the years following the European invasion.[6] Known to many as the "first wound," it was a physical, cultural, economic, and ecological genocide that haunts us to this day.*

The "New World" wasn't new at all. And yet Europe's "expansion" is not remembered as conquest but rather as exploration and discovery, its leaders hailed as heroes despite their horrific acts of violence and genocide. In the words of Dakota/Lakota Sioux writer and tribal attorney Ruth Hopkins, "It was crucial for European colonialists to paint Natives as aggressors to justify their own violence against the original inhabitants of this land. While Natives fought against settlers, these battles were waged primarily

---

* It is essential to learn the real history of the United States. Roxanne Dunbar-Ortiz has written many books on the history of Turtle Island from an Indigenous perspective, including *An Indigenous Peoples' History of the United States* and *Not a Nation of Immigrants*.

in self-defense. America invented the 'savage Indian' to subjugate Natives, abrogate Tribes' sovereign rights, and so they could freely initiate war against them for any reason whatsoever."[7]

The myth of separation, the justification of lies, and the assertion of violence to control, accumulate, and hoard wealth and power have been the underlying strategy of American expansion and progress. This tale of separation and superiority lives on today through militarism and economic domination.* The so-called war on terror that followed 9/11 was declared based on lies to advance a $21 trillion military operation that took nearly one million lives in the name of self-interest (not self-defense).[8] The last two decades have seen a growing culture of hypernationalistic state violence that is unprecedented. Democrats and Republicans alike have projected America's righteous cause of "expanding freedom and protecting human rights" as justification for a $725 billion defense budget to fund failed torture tactics, expansive drone killings, and an ever-growing carceral system.† The legacy of colonization continues today through economic and cultural imperialism that reaches across the globe, extending power over other countries and wreaking havoc on all of us. Meanwhile, our nation's leaders have neglected so much of what we really need. Militarism has only made climate instability worse and has not protected us from a pandemic that has killed an unfathomable amount in the US and around the world—that at its worst killed the same number of people as died on 9/11 every single day.

The goal of understanding where we come from and how we got here is not to get stuck in the realities of the past but to reckon with the consequences in our modern day. The paradigm of domination and conquest has been used throughout history to give governments and corporations unlimited access to natural land and resources, as well as dominion over people's bodies. It lives on not only through US foreign policy but in our

---

* Dr. Martin Luther King Jr. spoke of militarism as one of the "three evils" in his speech "Beyond Vietnam: A Time to Break the Silence."

† Check out Margaret Mead's essay "Warfare Is Only an Invention—Not a Biological Necessity." http://users.metu.edu.tr/utuba/Mead.pdf.

hearts and minds. And, thousands of years after its inception, on a sunny September day, that chaos came home.

Colonizer Virus

I am only now beginning to understand the colonizer within me. When I woke up to the real history of America, a rush of adrenaline rose up in me. I was moved, compelled to act, to channel energy toward fixing the past. I wanted to believe that colonization was a thing that other people did in some other time. I wanted to be angry and righteous about the bad things that bad people did. I wanted to prove that I was better. I wanted to be innocent, to be clean. Because the alternative was that I was complicit, that I was part of the problem. But it was my resistance to the truth that kept me stuck.

Colonization isn't just an event that happened in the past, it is a mindset that takes over the bodies, minds, and souls of its people. In *Decolonizing Wealth*, Indigenous activist and author Edgar Villanueva calls it the "colonizer virus"—referring to the infection that permeates every aspect of our culture and society and justifies domination and dehumanization. The virus enters the mind through the belief that one is separate from and supreme to everyone and everything around oneself. That belief allows the infection to thrive and grow until it has spread the disease throughout the whole system. From there the virus gets passed down through generations and "leads to ongoing acts of control and exploitation." Villanueva likened it to a "zombie invasion."[9]

Far from being a historical artifact, colonization continues on this land through the erasure of Indigenous history and present lived realities, treaties that continue to be broken and ignored, the theft of land by private corporations for drilling and mining, and the denial of democratic rights to US territories. American imperialism continues to build on the legacy of colonization abroad by assuming that the US is duty bound to share (force) our "advanced" society with (upon) others (through military might and economic coercion). US foreign policy—rooted in greed, power, and oil—has decimated nations, killed countless civilians, and left people more vulnerable than before. All of this stems from the idea that human beings are separate and superior to the environment we live in and depend on. It is a worldview that enables us to exploit natural resources and force species into extinction, to draw imaginary borders of belonging and call them nation-states, and to assume supremacy and domination over other human beings. Breaking from this mindset is critical to our survival.

Cultural appropriation and violence are offspring of colonization—an inherited attitude of entitlement that enables the stealing, glamorizing, and sterilizing of marginalized cultures. According to Susanna Barkataki, author of *Embrace Yoga's Roots*, it happens when a "dominant group in a position of privilege and power politically, economically or socially adopts, benefits from, shares and even exploits the customs, practices, ideas or social and spiritual knowledge of another, usually target or subordinate, society or people."[10] And, as I would soon learn, the wellness world is rife with it. Cultural appropriation is the commercialization of palo santo and sage to burn off bad energy, making these sacred plants less accessible to the people for whom they are cultural medicine. It is the overharvesting of quinoa to meet the ever-increasing demand for "superfoods" among foodies, making this staple unaffordable for the Andean people of Bolivia and Peru who have been living off the local grain for centuries. And it is the Westernization of yoga that is evangelized by white skinny devotees who neglect to honor and appreciate the people and cultures from which these practices originate, while profiting from its proliferation. The dehumanization of people, the corruption of spiritual tradition and practices, and the looting of Indigenous culture are the foundation that modern wellness is built upon. And until we confront these truths, we won't ever be well.

Many Indigenous worldviews teach that all life is interrelated and interdependent—that we coexist with all humans, nonhumans, and the planet. Colonization has attempted to eradicate this wisdom and convince us that we are separate. The myth of separation is at the heart of the lies we've been told and wounds we've incurred. It is the root of all suffering. Healing calls us to pick up the pieces, to recover the lost fragments of ourselves and our history, and to reclaim the whole truth of who we've always been, so that we can move toward an America that has never been (and is still possible).

Recovery

Nothing ever goes away until it teaches us what we need to know.

PEMA CHÖDRÖN

Nine days after 9/11 we piled into my living room—family, friends, neighbors—and leaned into the TV as President Bush addressed the nation. Our house had become mission control since the attacks—overcrowded with people, activated by the search, and stuffy with uncertainty and grief. We were yearning for answers: *How did this happen? What will make it right?* But when the president boldly declared retaliation—when he said "this will be a war like no other"—I flinched.[II] At the time, over 10,000 were still unaccounted for (including my stepdad). Hadn't we lost enough? Why would we put ourselves in a position of losing more? Of risking more lives? Of destroying more families? And in that moment, I had a punch to the gut—a knowing so deep it was undeniable—that meeting violence with more violence was not the answer. As I sat there feeling the sting of his words, the dread of what was to come, I knew that my life as I had known it was forever changed.

The heartbreak of what I lost on 9/11 was brutal. But equally painful was the realization that I had been living a lie. My all-American dream was to live in a safe community with good schools, to build a successful career and make lots of money, to have nice things. Everything I had come to know about what it meant to be well came crashing down with those towers. My perfectly curated "before" life was shattered, and the illusion that I was somehow insulated and sheltered from the rest of the world was destroyed. And despite society's attempts to deny us the truth, to numb our pain, to distract us, and to keep us separate and desperate, I was forever altered. Waking up to the truth of who we were as Americans, of who I was as an ignorant and complicit bystander, was excruciating and disorienting. And yet, seeing the lie of separation meant that I was seeing the truth of our connection, and there was no way in hell I was going back.

This kind of personal growth is not glamorous. It was a messy unraveling of everything I thought I knew, a constant questioning of the status quo and a relentless pursuit of the truth, so that I could birth a new way of being in the world. It is the detox and dismantling that are required for us to heal and emerge from the rubble. This kind of change doesn't happen all at once; it is a process. Sikh activist Valarie Kaur likens it to birth, asking, "What if this darkness is not the darkness of the tomb, but the darkness of the womb? What if our America is not dead but a country still waiting to be born? What if the story of America is one long labor?"[12]

9/11 was a symptom of a much larger disease that has been embedded in the fabric of this country. No longer can we cling to fantasy and protect our innocence; we must own up to our personal and collective responsibility. That means remembering the history of how we got here and speaking truthfully about the state of the world and the injustices that continue to pervade our culture. That means those of us who have inherited the colonizer virus doing our part to decolonize our minds from what we have internalized from our history and dismantle the systems that continue to uphold the culture of dominance. It means unhooking ourselves from our addiction to safety and control and embracing the vulnerability that is inherent in life. And it means engaging in a practice of truth and reconciliation that invites us to heal and repair the collective wounds of the past, so that we can allow for the possibility of the future.

Colonization and its modern offspring have led us to the brink of an apocalypse. Our survival depends on our willingness to do the opposite—to listen, learn, and follow the lead of Indigenous people.

Detoxing the Myth of Separation

In the days that followed 9/11, I found purpose in the desperate search for Joe. I scrambled for answers, plastered his face all over the city, bossed around anyone who would listen, as if I could manifest his rescue by sheer force. Taking charge was my drug, an adrenaline rush into an alternate reality that allowed me to escape the present moment and remain in the delusion that I could actually change things. I was unwavering in my effort. Until I was seated in the funeral home with my mom, trying to determine how to bury a body that wasn't there. And I lost my shit. It was as if my entire being was shouting, "No, I will not give up. I will not concede defeat and bury the possibility of his survival. I will not accept his death. I will not grieve the 2,973 people who are lost and waiting to be found. I will fix this." But there was no fixing 9/11. As I stormed out of the funeral home in a fury, something in me let go. As if holding it all together was my only way of holding onto hope.

Sometimes life pulls the rug out from under us. When that happens, our instinct is to cling, to find ground, to reach for something we can rely on. We scramble, we run, we do anything to escape the vulnerability and discomfort of what is. For me, it was the lie of separation and security that kept me fending for myself and minding my business. I curated my life in a safe and small bubble, insulated from everything and everyone around me. I thought I could control every outcome, defend every move, anticipate every next step. But it only left me more alone and isolated. Pema Chödrön says that "all addictions stem from this moment when we meet our edge and we just can't stand it."[13]

But difficult moments are also an invitation to courage. They are often the times when you realize that you can choose to do something different. Instead of conquering your fears, you move into relationship with them. When we learn to get comfortable with the uncomfortable, we are released from its grip. What might appear on the surface as chaos is actually freedom—freedom from the struggle against the fundamental ambiguity of simply being human. The one truth—the thing we know beyond a doubt—is that nothing is fixed and to be human is a dynamic experience that is ever changing. Permanence is a myth we buy into because we fear its opposite. The only way to get free is to let go.

What's left when we let go is vulnerability. Vulnerability calls us to connection. It acknowledges that we are not invincible. We are exposed. The practice of vulnerability is not neat and tidy, and yet it is powerful and profound. Cynthia Ocelli reminds us that the process of growth often looks like destruction. "The shell cracks, its insides come out and everything changes."[14] That was me. I was forced to disarm—to drop the protective shields I had built up around me, so that I could soften into the truth of what was happening and the grief of what was lost. For the first time in my life, I was exposed and undefended. Vulnerability demanded that I look pain squarely in the face and feel it.

No longer could I hide behind the veneer of strength and security. I had to reckon with my humanness—with how I was impacted and how I impacted others. I wasn't just a victim of a horrific event. I was both the wounded and the wounder. Coming to terms with my complicity in the culture and systems that led up to that moment was painful. I was ashamed that I had been unable to notice what was right in front of me or, worse, that I had chosen to look away. Grappling with my part and participation in America's racist colonial history not only implicated me in the dynamic system of oppression, but it also affirmed my belonging to the world—that I was part of something bigger than me, that I had a responsibility to the bigger "we," and that I could be a part of its healing. Learning to hold this paradox is how I was able to come back to the truth of our wholeness and interdependence.

When we feel separate, we experience the world through the lens of fear. Everyone and everything is suspect. We believe ourselves to be alone, solely responsible for our survival. We try to compensate for our lost sense of self by conquering and controlling our circumstances. The more we own, the more we control, the more secure we feel. We hoard, we compete, we judge, we oppress, we harm . . . all in the name of self-preservation. Recovering from the myth of separation requires that we embrace a vulnerability that speaks truth to power and moves toward healing and transformation. It invites us to go beyond personal responsibility and self-interest toward the messy, complex, and intersectional reality of who we really are in America and how we came to be here.

Every year on September 11 we are told to never forget. Society sponsors rituals and ceremonies to commemorate the memory of the almost 3,000 people who were lost on that day in 2001. We gather at firehouses, mourn in churches, and pay our respects at gravestones. But rarely are we asked to remember the millions of Indigenous lives sacrificed for the colonizer's cause. There is no holiday to acknowledge and grieve the millions of people in the Middle East killed in the so-called war on terror. The politics of memory is constructed and contrived. It is the story told by the people who benefit from it. But is that really remembering?

The opposite of remembering is *dismembering*, which means "to cut off or disjoin the limbs, members, or parts of."[15] Dismembering not only abandons whole truths about our past but also discards whole peoples in the process. It is not only the history of dispossession and genocide of Indigenous Peoples, it is the colonizer virus that continues to live on in our hearts and minds. It is the collective wound of separation that remains unhealed to this day—a wound that has been passed down through generations, from body to body, reenacting the old story of separation and domination. According to movement strategist and ecosystem designer Taj James, what keeps us stuck "is a fear born of forgetting."[16] Colonialism attempts to make us forget who we are and who we are to all living things. But not everyone has forgotten. Indigenous people carry with them the truth of their generational struggle and survival and the wisdom of our intrinsic relationship to all of life.*

Recognizing how we've been complicit in the myth of separation is essential to breaking from it. In moments of waking up, our temptation is to become so overwhelmed by guilt and shame that we withdraw and shut down. But that is exactly what the system of separation wants: for us to disengage and stay stuck and compliant. Compliance looks like going along to get along, conscious or unconscious negligence, avoiding conflict, and maintaining the status quo. But compliance doesn't, in fact, keep us safe and well. I spent most of my life on stolen land, occupying and extracting that which was not mine. But that wound would come back to haunt me on 9/11 when the ground was ripped out from under me. Leaning into the discomfort of who we are and how we got here is an invitation to become more enlivened by the awareness of interdependence. Fractured and separated is who we have become, but whole is who we have always been.

---

* For more on the work of decolonizing our hearts and minds, check out *Sacred Instructions* by Sherri Mitchell and *Braiding Sweetgrass* by Robin Wall Kimmerer.

If we don't acknowledge and account for the harms of the past, we will only reproduce them in the future. New, repackaged forms of domination and control are keeping us trapped in the past, unable to solve the problems of the present and create the future we all deserve. And if we build upon the pile of lies we've accumulated over the last 500 years, we will effectively seal our fate. Instead, we must break ground and excavate the truth so that we can work from a healthy foundation. Only when we face the hidden wounds and reclaim what has been lost can we move toward the personal and collective healing that we so desperately need.

Healing this moment requires first telling the truth about how we got here. History is a self-serving narrative shaped by people who are invested in it. It has been deliberately lost and rewritten by those in power who seek to control our understanding of reality and uphold systems of separation and hierarchy. Growing up, I was taught that Christopher Columbus was a hero who discovered America, when in actuality he was a greedy, genocidal man who was found lost at sea. I was encouraged to worship the Constitution as the sacred law of the land, despite the fact that it was written explicitly to exclude me and many others from its privileges. I learned that slavery ended with emancipation, when in fact it lives on today through the criminal system. Our refusal to face the truth of our collective traumas dooms us to perpetually reenact them. Penobscot activist and Indigenous rights attorney Sherri Mitchell writes that "a wound cannot be healed by pretending that it doesn't exist. It must be examined, cleansed, and tended. In order to create a healthy path forward, we must deal with the spiritual illness that plagues our past and present reality."[17]

I am the descendant of thirteen generations of colonizers. My paternal ancestor Edward Ketcham came over from Manchester, England, in 1635 as an indentured servant during the Puritan migration. He was designated a "freeman" a few years later, which gave him the right to vote and own land, and went on to live a prosperous life in New England that laid the groundwork for generations to come. I benefit from that legacy to this day. While I may feel far removed from my colonizer ancestors, their beliefs live on in me. They show up in how I occupy land and take up space without consideration for who else belongs there. In how I automatically assume control, ownership, or leadership in whatever work I am doing. In how I have taken other people's cultures and traditions without ever questioning whether I have a right to them. But knowing who I come from, regardless of the implications, is an essential part of detoxification. The wound of colonization has not just cut us off from each other but cut us off from parts of ourselves—the people and places we come from. Reclaiming our ancestry is rewriting the history of who we are in America and how we came to be here.

And we don't just come from people. We come from food and music, folklore and medicine. We come from land. We come from wisdom. But so much of that has been violently severed from its source, whether through colonization or the transatlantic slave trade. Indigenous Peoples and Black Americans have struggled to preserve the knowledge and wisdom that colonizers either stole or erased over time. My own immigrant ancestors gave in to the myth of the American Dream—trading in parts of themselves, their culture, and their religion in an attempt to fit in and belong to America. I've spent the last decade recovering my lineage, getting to know my ancestors, and reclaiming the medicine of the people I come from. Repairing our timelines is essential to disrupting the cycle of harm and healing the wound of colonization. By repairing the past we can build the future.

PERSONAL INQUIRY

I have learned to "sit with" myself in the mornings—sometimes on the mat, sometimes with a coffee, sometimes on the trail. Instead of jumping out of bed, I let myself unravel and unwind the night as I feel myself into a new day. I pay attention to what is waking inside of me, what wants to stretch open, what is tugging on my attention. And then I listen: What is stirring inside of me? What part of me is yearning to be felt? What is needed for healing? Where do I begin? I breathe into the questions not for answers but for witness. Acknowledging the pain, the tension, and the longing that lives in me and all around me is where I begin. From this place I can lean into and make space for essential questions.

- Who are the people that you come from?
- What have you inherited from colonization?
- What truths need to be recovered for personal and collective healing?
- What wounds need to be exposed and grieved?
- What is the medicine/ritual that you come from that will aid in healing the collective?
- What can you choose to do to disrupt the cycle of colonization?

Repairing the Past and Decolonizing the Present

It would have been easy for my story to end there. Girl wakes up, girl gets educated, girl heals her history, the end. But that just plays into the trap of the myth of separation. Reckoning with who we are and where we come from is not just a personal journey. It is a collective one. The truth of our interdependence demands that we not just decolonize our minds, but that we challenge the ideology of separation and the systems and structures that stem from it. The shared wound is one that cannot be addressed in isolation. Rather, it demands that we restore our relationship to each other and all things. And it affirms that we are all first responders on the front lines of healing.

Detoxing ourselves from the lies of separation, supremacy, and scarcity allows us to create new thought patterns and practices. For those of us who are not Native, it allows us to listen and appreciate Indigenous culture without romanticizing or appropriating its wisdom and ideas. It allows us to follow Indigenous activists and not assume leadership or control of the work. It urges us to respect that the land we occupy is not ours and honor its Native stewards. And it compels us to acknowledge our complicity and do what is necessary to repair the harms of the past. For people like myself, who are descended from white colonizers and continue to benefit from their legacy, our work is to become aware of the history that we come from and the land that we live on and reckon with the psychology of superiority that lives in us to this day. But it is also how we take action toward decolonization.

Decolonization is the rematriation of Indigenous land and resources. *Rematriation* means "returning the sacred to the Mother," in the words of the Indigenous-led *Rematriation* magazine.[18] It is not a denial of who we are and where we come from but rather a reckoning that invites us to tell the truth, repair past harms, and choose to do something different. Of course, we cannot simply "undo" the past and completely correct the taking of Indigenous lives and land. What we can do is take responsibility for our part. Decolonization is an everyday practice of changing our minds and taking action, actively rooting out and rejecting the colonized aspects of our institutions and culture. It means listening, learning and being accountable to Indigenous leaders advocating for Native sovereignty, self-determination, and rights, and redistributing power and resources to Indigenous communities on their terms.* And it means investing in truth, reconciliation, and reparations.

We repeat what we don't repair. It's a big reason we are still feeling the repercussions of colonialism in America, because we have not done the work of healing our collective wounds and repairing the harm done. We cannot simply leapfrog forward into positive social change and erase the past. We must invest in repair, restore our relationships, and make the changes necessary to transform our future. We can't truly know healing and reconciliation within ourselves until we face the wounds we have inherited, wounds we are a part of. Otherwise, we are doomed to

---

* Essential to our work is understanding what decolonization is (and isn't). The article "Decolonization Is Not a Metaphor" by Eve Tuck and K. Wayne Yang is a good source to help navigate this discourse: https://jps.library.utoronto.ca/index.php/des/article/view/18630.

perpetually reenact them. The truth and reconciliation process understands that reckoning with the past is necessary to transform experiences of conflict and harm into peace and connectedness. The "truth" part acknowledges that the United States was founded on genocide and slavery and seeks to create space for the voices of those most impacted, so that we can understand and address the needs of survivors. The "reconciliation" part imagines and designs new pathways of repair and reconstruction based on mutual respect and responsibility. Reconciliation is an ongoing and collective process.*

Healing the wound of separation is reclaiming all that is inherent to our wholeness, that has been lost and forgotten. Sherri Mitchell reminds us "we all carry the imprint of that wound in our souls."[19] And while our grief may be different based on how we've been impacted, it affirms the interconnected wound that binds us to each other and to the earth. I think that's why grief feels so overwhelming. Because collective grief cannot be separate from the collective. I cannot grieve 9/11 without grieving the first wound of colonization, just as I cannot grieve for the first responders without also grieving for all the people whose lives were taken in the war that followed. Grief is proof that we belong to each other. When we reach out to one another in times of grief, we are saying, "I can't do this alone, because I am not alone." By allowing ourselves to be seen in our whole truth and humanity and to receive love and support from others, we strengthen the ties that bind us and build more resilient possibilities for healing and community.

Grief also reminds us that we carry our ancestors with us, all those who came before and made it possible for us to be who we are today. Knowing who and where we come from allows us to both heal our timelines and bring forth the legacy of wisdom and learning that is essential to reconciling the past, meeting this moment, and creating a new future. We walk into a future of uncertainty with our ancestors at our backs and our hearts

---

* Fania Davis is a leading voice for truth and reconciliation and restorative justice in the US. Check out her book *The Little Book of Race and Restorative Justice: Black Lives, Healing, and US Social Transformation*.

broken open. Activist and writer Malkia Devich-Cyril shows us what's possible: "As we strip away the chains of nation-state to become true patriots to the nation that has not yet been born—the one beyond national borders and prison bars, the one forged in the fire of a deep, abiding love with an economy steeped in dignity and rights—we can come to know a richly resilient grief rather than a desperate, starving one."[20]

The myth of separation has brought us to the brink of extinction. Humans have made a mess of the world, and Mother Nature is unleashing her wrath upon us. We can no longer ignore the suffering that is all around us or deny the cost of extraction and exploitation on our planet. We must tell the truth and own up to our part. The collective wounds of the past have festered long enough. In remembering, we reclaim the lost parts of ourselves so that we can heal the whole. We call in the wisdom of our ancestors and ask them to walk with us on this path. We acknowledge that we come from great pain and suffering, and we come from great resilience and survival. And we actively engage in decolonizing ourselves and the systems we are a part of. Only then can we begin to recover what has been lost and move toward the wholeness and healing we are so desperately seeking.

COLLECTIVE PRACTICE: PROTECT THE SACRED

The myth of discovery that is taught in US schools and culture doesn't tell the whole story of the land currently called the United States. When colonizers happened upon the "New World," it wasn't new at all but home to thousands of years of history and advanced civilizations that rivaled the rest of the world's. For those of us who aren't Indigenous, learning whose land we reside on and the people who have stewarded the land for generations honors the truth of who we are and aims to correct the stories and practices that erase Indigenous Peoples, history, and culture.

Learn about the land and its people: Learn whose land you live on. Then go deeper: More than just the names of the original peoples of the land, what do you know of their lives and culture? What is the history of this land? How was the land used? And what do you know of the history that has shaped the land and its people and the challenges Indigenous people face today because of it?* Kanyon Sayers-Roods, a Mutsun Ohlone activist in Northern California, says, "The acknowledgement process is about asking, What does it mean to live in a post-colonial world? What did it take for us to get here? And how can we be accountable to our part in history?"[21]

Listen to the land stewards: The process of rematriation invites us to find out what local Indigenous organizers are calling for and following their lead.† For example, Sogorea Te' Land Trust, an urban Indigenous land trust, invites non-Native locals on Ohlone land in the San Francisco Bay Area to reimagine their relationship to the land and help return Indigenous land to Indigenous Peoples by building "many paths of radical reciprocity that are a part of rematriation and land return."[22] They also invite non-Native residents to pay a land tax out of respect for the sovereignty of Native people on their ancestral lands.‡ What are

---

* "Questions about 'Home'" from the Catalyst Project is an exercise for non-Native people to learn and reflect on the history and current struggles of Indigenous people and to reflect on the role of non-Native people in colonization and decolonization: https://collectiveliberation.org/wp-content/uploads/2018/10/Indigenous-Resistance-Homework.pdf.

† To learn more and support projects of rematriation and land return, check out the Sogorea Te' Land Trust: www.sogoreate-landtrust.org/rematriate-the-land-fund/.

‡ Honor tax is a way of paying reparations to the Indigenous nations who are stewards of the land that you reside on. Find out more from the Honor Tax Project at www.honortax.org.

Indigenous people in your community calling for? How can you answer the call from your particular social location?[23]

Protect the sacred: If you have access to land, wealth, and resources, consider your place in the lineage of theft and colonization and how you might contribute to repair and healing. Listen and learn from Indigenous Peoples' stories and knowledge. Recognize their leadership at the forefront and on the front line of climate change. And follow their lead as we work together to protect the sacred, repair the past, and engage in ecological restoration.*

---

* For Indigenous communities, the conservation of the environment is deeply intertwined with cultural preservation, land and water rights, tribal sovereignty, and the stewardship of ancestral homelands. Follow Indigenous-led organizations who are on the forefront of climate resilience, including Seeding Sovereignty, Indigenous Climate Action, Honor the Earth, and Indigenous Environmental Network.

CHAPTER 2

Seeking Healing

Life is a process of becoming, a combination of states we have to go through. Where people fail is that they wish to elect a state and remain in it. This is a kind of death.

ANAÏS NIN

Broken.

I remember standing on the corner of 48th and 8th. The light changed but I was unable to move. It had been like this for days since the funeral. A funeral that offered absolutely no closure in a never-ending search for answers, for body parts, for meaning. They got their ceremonious send-off, and now we were left with this mess.

A cabbie honked his horn—a sign of things gone back to normal. It was business as usual again in NYC. Whatever specialness existed in the aftermath was replaced by rush hour and a relentless drive to move on. Everyone had moved on. And yet I couldn't move.

The fight and fire that fueled my adrenaline for weeks after 9/11 was extinguished. And I missed it. The drive to find Joe, to find answers, gave me purpose. My anger felt valid, satisfying even. But now I was just a shell of my former self. Reduced to rubble like those buildings. I didn't have words at the time for what I was experiencing. It wasn't just my world turned upside down, it was a complete unraveling of my body, mind, and spirit.

The brokenness felt intolerable, something to be avoided at all costs, to be hidden and anesthetized. I was desperate for relief, for distraction, for comfort. I became addicted to anything and everything that offered me an escape from the pain. Drinking, drugs, work, and working out were my go-tos for simply getting through each day. I learned to look forward to numb. Numb was doable, reality was not.

The people around me couldn't handle it either. They assured me it was going to be OK. They sent me to psychiatrists. They encouraged medication. They bought me nice things, fed me drinks, took me out. Good intentions designed not just to make it better but to make it go away. My suffering was not just intolerable to me, it was intolerable to everyone.

I was aware that I no longer fit into that system. It didn't accommodate brokenness. It demanded that I get back to normal. But I started to question if there was even a "normal" to get back to. It felt impossible to go on as before.

So, I channeled all of my suffering and grief into my quest to find a cure for my pain.

Sick Care

I'm the proud daughter of a nurse and the descendant of a long line of women healers. Whenever I was feeling sick when I was growing up, there was always a remedy at the ready. The women of my family were always trading secrets and conspiring to heal. They embodied the spirit of care with a splash of intervention—always willing to proxy as a midwife, pediatrician, pharmacist, or hospice worker. This is the folklore that I come from, a system of community care that is by and for the people. But in recent years, our family's wisdom has taken a back seat to the medical industry's fast fixes and pharmaceuticals.

We live in a society that encourages instant relief, quick satisfaction, and distractions as antidotes to pain. It focuses on symptoms rather than root causes, emphasizes treatment rather than prevention, hands out simple cures for complex conditions, and relies heavily on drugs. What society considers "medicine" today is rooted in allopathy (meaning "other than disease") and is grounded in the use of medications or surgery to treat or suppress disease. It is a system that waits until we have become sick before it kicks into action. It is not concerned with preventing health problems by creating the conditions for bodies to thrive, but rather with detecting, diagnosing, and treating disease. It invests in what's wrong with us at the expense of strengthening our bodies' own defenses and abilities to heal themselves. And it's become completely unsustainable. Six out of ten Americans are suffering from a chronic disease, and while treatment for chronic diseases makes up 90 percent of healthcare spending, the investment in prevention only amounts to 2.9 percent.[1]

We don't have a system of healthcare in this country; we have a system of sickcare. What's worse is that it's driven by a massive industry that not only profits from our sickness but is motivated by profit. Treatment does not follow scientific health guidelines but the logic of a voracious and unregulated market. It sells us wildly expensive drugs and fancy treatment plans but rarely addresses the root causes, which only puts people in a perpetual cycle of dependency and debt. Meanwhile, the US spends nearly one-fifth of its gross domestic product on healthcare (more than $3 trillion a year, which is equivalent to the entire economy of France) and delivers worse outcomes and sicker people than any other industrialized country.[2] As Wendell Berry writes, "What is wrong with us contributes more to the 'gross national product' than what is right with us."[3] Nevertheless, we find ourselves spending hand over fist to get healthy and happy.

Not only is it more profitable to treat diseases than to prevent them, but a lot of money can be made from healthy people who believe they are sick. This sort of "disease mongering" promotes the expansion of treatable illness through the medicalization of ordinary life in order to expand markets for those who sell and deliver treatments.[4] Pharmaceutical companies are actively involved in making up diseases, convincing people that they have them, and then marketing treatments to both prescribers and consumers. This trend dates back to 1879 when Listerine saw an opportunity to market an over-the-counter mouthwash to the general public. But they needed a disease to match their "cure." So they made one up: halitosis, a manufactured diagnosis for bad breath to increase demand for a solution.[5] Disease mongering lives on today to validate the many "disorders" (and profitable solutions) we are being sold. But it is also how we pathologize the behavior and life choices of anyone who doesn't fit into dominant cultural standards. All of this is a social construct among individuals, institutions, systems, corporations, and politicians that exists to make money and keep people sick and dependent.

When companies are not making up diseases, they're exploiting them. Big Pharma spends more money on advertising than it does on research and development (it is illegal to market to consumers in every other country except New Zealand), invests more in government lobbying than any other industry, and pays doctors over $3 billion per year to push their prescriptions.[6] Take OxyContin, the popular drug from Purdue Pharma that is closely linked to the opioid epidemic. Purdue launched the drug with what many would call marketing fraud. They misrepresented the effects, insisting it was more effective and less addictive, and drove sales by targeting and incentivizing physicians. By 2001 sales were soaring, and by 2014 deaths from opioid overdoses had quadrupled.[7] In 2016 alone, an estimated 64,000 Americans died of opioid overdoses—more than the combined death tolls for Americans in the Vietnam, Afghanistan, and Iraq wars.[8]

Of course, none of this functions without the unquestionable authority of the doctor, who remains predominantly male. While women make up a majority of healthcare workers in the US (80 percent), most of the leaders (senior executives, CEOs, decision makers) are men.[9] But that is not how it's always been. For centuries, women were doctors without degrees. They were the people's healers—midwifing babies, prescribing herbs, and nursing the sick and wounded. Many of the remedies discovered by women healers are still being used today in modern medicine. Women healers used willow bark to treat inflammation, the essence of which informed a key compound in aspirin. They used garlic to treat ulcers, an antidote proven and prescribed to this day to lower cholesterol and help block platelet formation (blood clots). But as the church-state emerged, women healers became a threat to people in power. In *Witches, Midwives, and Nurses*, Barbara Ehrenreich and Deirdre English note that "the suppression of women health workers and the rise to dominance of male professionals was not a 'natural' process . . . it was an active takeover,"[10] which resulted in women being mocked, abused, and burned at the stake. Witch hunts were an organized campaign by the church and state against women healers (and peasant uprisings).* And by the nineteenth century, white men in medicine had professional dominion over the human body. It was in that context that the word *normal* emerged to differentiate between who gets to be well and who doesn't.

The "Science" of Normal

I won the lottery at birth. Born white, nondisabled, cisgender, and middle-class, I was always at the front of the line, well-liked by other kids, rewarded by teachers and adults. I played the part that was assigned to me. No one told me the rules. I figured it out along the way by paying attention to who wins and who loses, who gets picked first on the softball field and who is the last one standing, who gets ridiculed and who gets to just be, who gets favored in class and who gets forgotten, who gets to belong and who gets left out. I fell on the lucky side of that equation growing up, but not everyone did.

This rift between who gets to belong and who doesn't didn't come out of nowhere. When modern medicine emerged in the 1800s as the authority over the human body, so did the concept of "normal."[11] Defined as average, ideal, and functional, normal became the standard that would divide and distinguish between good and bad. While who is considered normal has morphed over time, it has most often excluded those with physical and cognitive differences, gender-nonconforming people, and anyone who isn't white. Everything and anything that diverged from the construction of normal was deemed

---

* Learn more about the history and persecution of women healers in *Witches, Midwives, and Nurses: A History of Women Healers* by Barbara Ehrenreich and Deirdre English, *Voodoo Queen: The Spirited Lives of Marie Laveau* by Martha Ward, and *Witch: Unleashed. Untamed. Unapologetic.* by Lisa Lister.

abnormal. These "scientific" judgments were drawn from an imported Euro-colonial history that included the separation, torture, and killing of anyone who was seen as "different." And they played a major role in validating the idea that many social ills of the time were caused by the proliferation of the wrong sort of people. The intervention that followed was eugenics.

Eugenics, the idea that the human population can be improved through selective breeding, was originally developed by Francis Galton, inspired by his cousin Charles Darwin and the theory of natural selection. Scientists like Galton, with strong biases about who was fit and unfit, weaponized science to substantiate a hierarchy of humans and drive social policies and technological interventions designed to create a "superior race."[12] This desire for racial perfection through eugenics programs found fertile ground in America and became the ideological underpinnings of state-sponsored discrimination, forced sterilization, and genocide. It supported the myth that social inequalities stem from biological differences, blaming those marginalized by structural inequality for their disadvantages. Thus began the disturbing resilience of eugenics that has shaped culture and politics ever since.*

Theories of the genetic inferiority of certain social groups went hand-in-hand with race-making in America. In the nineteenth century, Samuel Morton, known as the father of scientific racism, would posit that cranial capacity determined intellectual ability (known as craniometry) and apply this analysis to support a racial classification that put "Caucasians" (a term that was used to refer to Europeans from a particular region) on the top rung and "Negroes" (referring to the physical features of a group of people rather than where they originated) on the bottom.[13] This pseudoscience reinforced the false idea that there are genetically different human races and would be used to justify chattel slavery and the exploitation, experimentation on, and abuse of people of color.†

---

* For more on the history and resilience of scientific racism in research and medicine, check out *Medical Apartheid* by Harriet Washington and *Superior: The Return of Race Science* by Angela Saini.

† It wasn't until 1998 that the American Anthropological Association issued a statement on race, concluding that contemporary science makes clear that human populations are not "unambiguous, clearly demarcated, biologically distinct groups."

Eugenics, meaning well-born, isn't just the promotion of well-being and reproduction of the "superior race." It is also population control and violent strategies to discourage and prevent the reproduction of those deemed "undesirable." Building on the rapid institutionalization in the late 1800s and early 1900s, those who were deemed "unfit"—poor women, people with physical or mental disabilities, and anybody who was considered sexually deviant—were committed, nonconsensually sterilized, and prevented from reproducing. A system of targeted and forced sterilization was passed into law in thirty-two states, impacting between sixty and seventy thousand people, and in 1927 the Supreme Court upheld a state's right to forcibly sterilize a person considered "unfit" to procreate (mostly because of perceived mental illness, but also due to disabilities, poverty, and/or race), claiming that "three generations of imbeciles is enough."[14] In the mid-twentieth century, efforts to fight formal segregation led to anxiety about maintaining a white majority, and coerced sterilization became increasingly targeted at Black, Puerto Rican, Mexican, and Native American women (25 percent of whom were sterilized by 1976).[15] Immigration restrictions would be used to control who comes into the country, and sterilization to prevent those already here from procreating. The eugenics project in the US was so robust that the Nazis are said to have borrowed it from us.

But theories of genetic inferiority didn't stop by the end of the twentieth century; they simply morphed. What was once an overt optimization of the gene pool has become a much more subversive weapon assigning value and blame to different populations. It is present in a prison system that continues to enforce reproductive control among the incarcerated. It has shaped immigration policy over time, applying quotas to "less desirable" nationalities, banning immigrants from certain countries, and separating families. It plays into the dismantling of welfare and cuts to the social safety net that disadvantage the poor. And it is alive in a culture and system that upholds some bodies as valuable and normal and oppresses and discards others.

In *The Body Is Not an Apology* Sonya Renee Taylor reminds us that we live in a world of default bodies. "The default body becomes the template for the normal body," she writes, which in turn makes everything else different, undesirable, and dangerous.[16] We become indoctrinated into a system and culture that organizes, judges, and ranks bodies according to who is most able, most productive, most conforming, and most desirable. This manifests in what Taylor refers to as "body terrorism": the historical and contemporary violence associated with body hatred—our own and others'—and the devastating impacts that come with that. "All this is fueled by a system that makes large quantities of money off our shame and bias," she shares.[17] But who decides what is normal? And to what end?

According to writer, abolitionist, and community organizer Mia Mingus, "The Medical Industrial Complex is an enormous system with tentacles that reach beyond simply doctors, nurses, clinics, and hospitals. It is a system about profit, first and foremost, rather than 'health,' well-being and care. Its roots run deep and its history and present are connected to everything including eugenics, capitalism, colonization, slavery, immigration, war, prisons, and reproductive oppression."[18] In other words, it is the invisible hand that controls bodies and calls it health. The medical-industrial complex is driven by purpose: to designate and reinforce superiority, to manage access to care and treatment, to control populations through medicalization and institutionalization of those deemed abnormal and disposable, and to define desirability and the moral code of health. Of course, none of this is mutually exclusive and all of it colludes to rank bodies and drive profitability. Now whole industries grossing billions of dollars are built on the concepts of "normal" and "abnormal" and on the ideas of "well" and "disordered."*

When contemplating who decides what is "normal" and "healthy" in modern medicine, we need only look back at history and the hand of white patriarchy, Christian domination, and, eventually, capitalism that has benefited ever since. It is how alternative modalities and anything outside the mainstream of medicine have been discredited and labeled as "pseudoscience." It's boardrooms of men legislating forced birth. It's the pathologization of queer and trans lives. It is the refusal to insure people with

---

* Check out this thorough mapping of the US medical-industrial complex by Mia Mingus, Patty Berne, Cara Page, and a number of other disability and healing justice thinkers: https://leavingevidence.wordpress.com/2015/02/06/medical-industrial-complex-visual/.

preexisting conditions. It is scientific experimentation on people of color. It is the dehumanization of people with disabilities. It is Big Pharma and the so-called war on drugs. And it is the incarceration of people deemed "criminal" and "mentally disabled." All in the name of "health."

Health as a Moral Imperative

Health is often defined as "the absence of any disease or impairment." But that is not the understanding that I grew up with. I saw "health" in skinny bodies and clear complexions, in dynamic workouts and low-fat meals, in happy faces and positive outlooks. I learned that health was popularity, achievement, and status. And that is exactly how we've come to understand health in modern culture—a one-size-fits-all prescription for the perfect body, which ultimately means the most "normal" body.

Robert Crawford coined the term *healthism* in 1980 to describe this ideology, which believes that health is the sole responsibility of the individual and judges people's worth according to their perceived health.[19] Healthism is the idea that anyone who isn't "healthy" or "normal" just isn't trying hard enough. It can be seen in the ways folks judge bigger-bodied people as if they have committed some crime against culture's idea of "good health." Simultaneously, those who choose deprivation (dieting) or indulgence (Botox) in the name of health are praised as morally superior. But it's not enough to try and live up to the expectations of healthism; we're shamed for it. Social media is full of trolling disguised as care or concern and, above all, desiring and protecting the perfect body at all costs. I myself have fallen into this trap time and time again—striving for the impossible, starving my body, comparing, competing, and climbing the ladder of "health" only to fall into a shame spiral for failing to live up to society's unrealistic expectations.

In their book *Against Health: How Health Became the New Morality*, Jonathan Metzl and Anna Kirkland warn against this toxic culture of health, arguing that far too often health rhetoric advances value judgments, assumptions, and hierarchies that have much more to do with power and privilege than well-being.[20] Healthism protects the status quo. It leads to victim blaming and internalized oppression. Even the discourse over healthcare is centered around the individual's achievements and failures in optimizing their bodies. Before the Affordable Care Act, insurance companies routinely denied healthcare to people with preexisting conditions (the very people who needed it most).[21] Basically, if you get sick, it's your fault.

All of which ignores the evidence-based consensus that social determinants of health—things like poverty, racism, and violence—influence our well-being far more than individual behaviors.[22] But the disconnect between the evidence around social determinants and our obsession with changing individual health behaviors is important, because healthism only thrives in a system where the dominant groups do not have to grapple with things like hunger, war, poverty, and discrimmination as a part of their health regimen. Personal responsibility around health is only possible for the privileged—those not subject to the very real health disparities that exist today. Healthism is often targeted at the most vulnerable. Women have historically been gaslit by the medical industry that attributed their health claims to "hysteria" and hormones. Black people are nutrition-shamed for having higher rates of diabetes, despite the evidence that correlates the disease to systemic food and housing insecurity. And poor immigrant communities have been blamed for the spread of infectious disease when the lack of social support and healthcare is almost always to blame. While mainstream culture continues to point the finger at those who are sick, personal choice is not to blame for our biggest health crises. Inequality is.

Those of us indoctrinated into healthism are so preoccupied by our own personal health struggles—from illness to fatigue to anxiety to gut issues—that we don't see the larger socio-environmental system our problems are rooted in. When I think back to all the energy I've invested obsessing about my weight or my acne or my anxiety or my insecurity, it's no wonder I didn't see the bigger problems. I was too distracted. But when we pretend that social and natural environments have nothing to do with our health outcomes, we believe ourselves to be in control of our choices and "empowered" in our morality and judgments around what it means to be healthy. And in doing so, we uphold the system that not only separates the individual from their environment but benefits from our complicity. But in this context, are we really well?

The Culture of Cure

After 9/11 I struggled to get back to "normal." Normal was getting over it and moving on as if nothing had happened. But something *had* happened and I was forever altered. Depression kept me stuck and sick, isolated and excluded. After the attention of 9/11 faded away, so did my friends and my community. It became clear to me that this deviation—the abnormal—was not welcome or accepted. Not only did I feel broken, but I was deemed broken by the culture around me—a thing to be fixed and cured.

But the idea that any one of us is an object to be fixed or cured *is* the problem. It's how we over-pathologize the human condition to warrant medical or mental health intervention. Under the fifth edition of the *Diagnostic and Statistical Manual of Mental Disorders* (*DSM-5*, the latest version of the diagnostic statistical manual issued by the American Psychiatric Association and the primary handbook used by healthcare professionals in the US), temper tantrums could be diagnosed as disruptive mood dysregulation disorder, grief could be diagnosed as major depression, and first-time substance abusers could be diagnosed with substance use disorder.[23] The authority of diagnosis is incredibly powerful. At its best, diagnosis can provide clarity and specificity, peace of mind, and access to vital medical technology. At its worst, it can shame, devalue, and pathologize people, especially when it is used to declare someone as incompetent, thus stripping them of their right to make decisions for themselves (and historically resulting in removal, isolation, restraint, neglect, violence, and death). For many, diagnosis is messy in how it often carries stigma and how it often is required to receive the medical and social support needed to survive.

Hand in hand with diagnosis is the concept of disorder. Words like *disorder*, *defect*, *deficiency* are qualifications, and they are judgments that imply more than their prefixes' "apart and away from." They categorize people as "wrong, broken, and in need of repair" and set up the system to exclude, discriminate, and devalue entire communities and cultures from what is considered worthy of health and well-being. The historical pathologization of LGBTQ adults and children—branding them as "ill" and "deviant" based on their sexual orientation, gender identity, or gender expression—is an example of this and has been used to justify subjecting LGBTQ people, even at young ages, to forced or coercive psychiatric evaluations, hormone therapy, surgeries, and even sterilization. The associated stigma also shaped how the US responded to the HIV/AIDS crisis, resulting in lack of funding, denial of care and treatment, and widespread discrimination. It was not until 1987 that the American Psychiatric Association fully removed homosexuality from the *DSM*, and despite several revisions to the diagnosis for transgender people, being trans is still considered a psychological disorder to be cured rather than a natural human variation to be valued.[24]

Where there is diagnosis, there must be cure. Cure is embedded in a Western medical system designed to disregard self and community determination and foster medical authority over everyone's bodies and minds. Cure upholds the idea that "health" is synonymous with normalcy. We find cure in dieting and weight loss surgery. We find cure in skin lightening creams marketed to women of color. We find cure in reparative therapy promising to change one's sexual orientation. Cure is not just about medical research, it's an ideology. "Cure rides on the back of normal and natural. Insidious and pervasive. It impacts most of us," says Eli Clare, author of *Brilliant Imperfection*. "In response, we need neither a wholehearted acceptance nor an outright rejection of cure—but rather a broad-based grappling."[25] Cure is a contradictory mess.

But cure is not neutral in an ableist world. Leah Lakshmi Piepzna-Samarasinha, author of *Care Work: Dreaming Disability Justice*, says, "Ableism believes that when there's something 'wrong' with a body and or mind, the only desirable outcome to that wrongness is cure. It also believes that you can either be fixed or broken—there's nothing in between."[26] And of course ableism is made even more complicated by race, class, gender, immigration status, sexuality, age, and so on.* Disability exists in a dimension beyond

---

* The Movement for Black Lives breaks down how the medical-industrial complex is rooted in anti-Blackness and how to "end the war on Black health and Black disabled people." https://m4bl.org/policy-platforms/end-the-war-black-health/.

what is perceived as "normal." Normal assumes that everyone is abled, and designs society accordingly. Everyone else is an afterthought, an other-thought, an invisible thought. But access to normal is unpredictable and precarious, even for those who are nondisabled.

. I only ever understood disability as something that happens to other people. Until it happened to me. It was a few years after 9/11 and I was on holiday in Queenstown, New Zealand. I had always been active, athletic, and adventurous and decided to go horseback riding one afternoon. It was a beautiful and leisurely ride through the backcountry, until my horse got spooked, galloped for about fifty yards, and then bucked me ten feet into the air. After thirty excruciating minutes on the ground, unable to move, I was able to stand up with the help of others. Almost immediately, I knew that my body would never be the same and would eventually discover that I had broken my back. But as I would soon find out, my body wasn't the problem. Rather, it was that I no longer fit into a society designed for able bodies.

For me, disability wasn't in the chronic pain I experience to this day, nor the inability to sit or stand or walk for long periods of time, nor in being unable to carry bags while shopping or traveling, nor losing feeling and function in my right arm. It existed in all the places I couldn't go, all the activities I couldn't engage in. And it existed in my isolation. The privilege that I'd experienced for most of my life had not only oriented me to see access and convenience as normal, but it completely invisibilized the experience that one in five Americans have when they're confronted by a system that is designed to ignore and exclude them. Disability is not located in the individual's body and mind but in the world. It is a construct: a product of a toxic culture that defines normal in the form of beauty, performance, productivity, and obedience.

The wellness industry only reinforces this dynamic. It lures people in by promising individual health without acknowledging the conditions that cre-ated our suffering in the first place. It reinforces ideas of normal by dangling images of white, skinny, flexible, cisgender women in tight-fitting clothes and muscled, white, cisgender men in front of our eyes. It praises "sweat" and high-intensity workouts that exclude disabled bodies as the pinnacle of well-ness performance. It is an entire business model built on the idea that we are not good enough and in need of a fix. "Mainstream ideas of 'healing' deeply believe in ableist ideas that you're either sick or well, fixed or broken, and that nobody would want to be in a disabled or sick or mad bodymind," writes Piepzna-Samarasinha. "These ableist ideas often carry over into healing spaces that call themselves 'alternative' or 'liberatory.' The healing may be acupuncture and herbs, not pills and surgery, but assumptions in both places abound that disabled and sick folks are sad people longing to be 'normal,' that cure is always the goal, and that disabled people are objects who have no knowledge of our bodies."[27] But this only reduces us to fragmented versions of ourselves, pigeonholed and prodded into unhuman ways of being in the world. Challenging normative ideas of health and well-being requires that we reclaim our wholeness and recognize that the only thing abnormal and diseased are the systems we are a part of.*

---

* Understanding ableism and disability justice is essential to our personal and collective healing. Check out *Care Work: Dreaming Disability Justice* by Leah Lakshmi Piepzna-Samarasinha, *Brilliant Imperfection: Grappling with Cure* by Eli Clare, *Disability Visibility: First Person Stories from the Twenty First Century* edited by Alice Wong, *All the Weight of Our Dreams: On Living Racialized Autism* edited by Lydia X. Z. Brown, E. Ashkenazy, and Morénike Giwa Onaiwu, and *Spectrums: Autistic Transgender People in Their Own Words* edited by Maxfield Sparrow.

Recovery

All bodies are unique and essential. All bodies are whole.
All bodies have strengths and needs that must be met. We
are powerful not despite the complexities of our bodies,
but because of them. We move together, with nobody left
behind. This is disability justice.

SINS INVALID

I never identified with being a survivor. I was a fighter and a fixer. I had already survived many things in my life. I had survived childhood divorce by learning how to fend for myself. I had survived family alcoholism by becoming a peacemaker. I had survived date rape by eating and drinking away the shame. And I had survived the death of loved ones by throwing myself back into work. I was rehearsed in the practice of plowing through—relentless, insidious, and unstoppable in my attempt to cope and return to normal. But I was tired of escaping and barely surviving. So I set out on a desperate search for healing. For months I cycled through medical treatments, psychotherapies, and spiritual rituals, until I unexpectedly found it on the mat.

I dragged myself to yoga for all the wrong reasons—it was the latest trend to whip your body into shape and had the added benefit of calming your mind. On one particular day in November 2001, I planned to hit it hard, to beat down and sweat out the despair. But something else happened. As I moved and breathed on my mat, I started to feel . . . everything. My body began to unravel and with it my pain, my fear, and my loss. And it sucked. But it was the most real thing I had felt in a long time. Something was happening to me. While I didn't have words for it at the time, I could feel myself changing—falling apart and falling back together again. And I realized, right there on my mat, that all my efforts to fix myself were just a desperate attempt to get back to normal, to return to the "before" state. But healing isn't linear or transactional. It demands that we go through the pain and suffering and come completely undone first. Only then can we remember and reconnect to the part of us that has been whole all along.

Finding my practice was like coming home again. It was the first time in a long time I was able to experience myself all at once—all my grief, my pain, my suffering alongside and simultaneous with my joy, my vulnerability, and my deep yearning. I let myself be not who the world needed me to be, not the "put together" version of me, not even the fixed and cured version of me, but rather the me that was heartbroken, traumatized, and stuck. And it was in that place, in the messy middle, that I discovered that healing was possible, and it was unlike anything I had ever known before.

Healing is not what they are selling us. It is an inside-out process of recovery that conspires to return us to wholeness. We are not a *thing* to be fixed. We are whole human beings who deserve to thrive on our terms. Detoxing from the culture of healthism and normativity is reclaiming our right to heal. It has nothing to do with someone else's idea of normal; instead it meets us where we are and values our whole selves. Recovery is an embodied practice that helps us remember and reclaim all parts of ourselves as we move toward our own self-determined expression of health. It is a whole-system approach to healing that acknowledges we are only as well as the systems around us, and it demands that we challenge the medical-industrial complex and imagine new ways of caring for each other.

Unlearning Ideas of Broken and Fixed

Society would have you believe that you have no power, that you are helpless in the face of stress and dis-ease. It tells us to "just deal with it," giving us products and tools to distract, isolate, and alleviate our discomfort. It doles out drugs and diagnoses, breakthrough treatments and cutting-edge therapies, all for the sake of a controlled outcome and supposed cure. But there is no health discovery or scientific innovation that can prevent people from experiencing painful things or erase their need for support. Despite what they tell you, healing is rarely found in some miracle cure or ground-breaking drug. Healing is an inside game.

But that's not what we're taught. I grew up believing that so-called health was something you purchased, or a pill you took, or a service you subscribed to. That my body was not to be trusted, but something to be tamed, manipulated, and controlled. In school I learned how to read and write, but not how to move through change or navigate adversity or respond to threats. I developed the ability to suppress my feelings, to numb, to seek pleasure and avoid pain. All of which kept me grasping outside of myself for some semblance of health and normalcy. But that's not healing. Writer and facilitator adrienne maree brown says that "healing is the resilience instinct of our bodies, a skill we unlearn as we are taught to pay for and rely on data and medicine outside of our own awareness to be well."[28] No one is going to do the healing for you.

Only when I went inward and started to listen to my body did I really start to know myself. My body is memory, imprinted by all it has come in contact with. It is the abandoned little girl whenever I experience rejection. It is the assaulted woman whenever I am walking down a deserted street. It is the cautious family member whenever I'm around an alcoholic. It is the grieving New Yorker whenever I'm walking through the remnants of downtown Manhattan. Each time my body remembers, I am thrown. Made aware of borders that surround me by the encroachment itself. These imprints accumulate like badges, shaping me into the defended and suspicious person I have become. I carry them with me, like a passenger in a car. Wherever I go, my wounding comes with me, helping me navigate danger and make sense of the world around me. It senses, before I do, the threat or injustice and moves to act. It is my irrational survivor and my fiercest advocate. And all of it has been necessary for me to be who I am today.

To understand healing, we must understand our trauma. According to Staci Haines, a leader in the field of somatics, trauma is "an experience, series of experiences, and/or impacts from social conditions, that break or betray our inherent need for safety, belonging, and dignity."[29] But the experience and shaping of trauma is not the event itself but our ability to recover from it. Psychologist Peter Levine, founder of Somatic Experiencing, calls it "incomplete physiological responses suspended in fear."[30] Trauma hijacks our brains, preventing us from responding to fear in balanced and compassionate ways. It is unrelenting and ubiquitous, never letting up or giving its subjects a chance to recover. As a result, we become disconnected. Why? "Because it's too painful to be ourselves," says renowned addiction expert Gabor Maté.[31]

But trauma is not just individual experiences. It's the way people are harmed by systems rooted in inequality and injustice that perpetually threaten their sense of safety and belonging, like a criminal justice system that targets Black and Brown men or a misogynist culture that objectifies women and girls. Oppression is trauma. It is a history of pain and suffering that blows through one generation to the next when uninterrupted. Epigenetics has shown us that trauma and extreme stress such as poverty, violence, and discrimination can live on many generations later, impacting our ability to relate, respond, and thrive.

Trauma causes a fragmentation of the self—a compartmentalization of experiences, a dissociation from the psyche, and the development of strategies designed to cope and return to "normal." Although we may survive trauma, our suffering comes from an inability to fully process and discharge the energy associated with it, pulling us apart from ourselves and one another. Along with it comes the shame of our struggle and survival, that we have become damaged and broken in the process. These experiences and patterns imprint themselves onto us, shaping our identity, behaviors, relationships, and worldview. But it doesn't stop there. When trauma is not transformed, it is often transferred. And until we break the cycle and heal the wounds of our life and lineage, we will further a culture of trauma where hurt people hurt people.*

Healing begins with acknowledging that we are impacted by traumatic experiences and social conditioning. Not only does this awareness allow us to recognize our survival-shaping when it is happening, but it also opens up the possibility for new embodied patterns that give us the sense

---

* Here are some resources on trauma that I've found helpful: *The Body Keeps the Score* by Bessel van der Kolk, *Peace from Anxiety* by Hala Khouri, *The Politics of Trauma* by Staci Haines, and *Restorative Yoga for Ethnic and Race-Based Stress and Trauma* by Gail Parker.

of safety, dignity, and belonging we are yearning for. When I discovered this for myself, I was able to notice when I went into survival mode and choose to do something else. I could bear witness to two very different and valid parts of me with clarity and compassion: the part of me that is a survivor who needs to protect herself from harm, and the part of me that is an advocate who understands that my survivor is doing the best she can given the circumstances. Healing does not require that we deny or dispose of the parts of ourselves that are hurting and imperfect; rather, it requires us to include, integrate, and even embrace them. There is no right way to heal. There is just remembering our whole selves.

But modern medicine doesn't sell us wholeness, it sells us "normal." Normal is the predominant context that we live in, always operating in the background of our systems and choices. It is a consummate shape-shifter, masking itself in scientific discovery, medical innovation, and even wellness trends—all for the sake of fixing what is deemed as broken or different. And it doesn't just exist out in the world. It manifests within us. Many of us internalize society's ideas of normal, healthy, and able until they become something we've bought into, something we strive for. Disability, on the other hand, is framed as sad, lacking, and undesirable—something to be avoided and pitied. Our compliance reinforces the system that controls who gets to be normal, included, resourced, and uplifted. Detoxing from a culture that favors nondisabled bodies and minds calls us to challenge these dominant ideas of normal that see disabled people as "other" and treat disability as a pathology. Divergent and diverse states have always existed in nature. Healing invites us to bring our bodies back into the conversation. All bodies— bodies that are different, bodies that have limitations, bodies that fall outside of what is considered normal—are worthy of thriving.

Practices like yoga, meditation, mindfulness, and somatics that focus on the interaction between body, mind, and behavior help us build our awareness of the body's biological, mental, and emotional processes. Instead of reacting to immediate sensations and symptoms, we're encouraged to pause, go deeper, and explore what's underneath the surface, where it may have come from, and what is needed. We are invited to move through our discomfort—not around or away from it. When we can be in relationship to it, we can gain more insight into how to work with it. Society teaches us to reject suffering—to numb, avoid, distract, and work around our uncomfortable feelings. It pathologizes discomfort and disorientation as things to be erased rather than confronted. But any attempt to bypass discomfort only amplifies it. The only way is through. If we can learn to trust and respect the body's inherent resilience and ability to know itself and heal itself, we can make better choices for health and healing on our terms. Resilience is our nature.

On my yoga mat, I was able to experience discomfort and disorientation in small, manageable ways. It was a training ground to develop the tools and capacity to respond when things—either pleasant or painful—came up in my body. I would witness my inner fighter emerge when confronted with sensation or limitation, my conditioned tendency to push through, to conquer even, to figure it out. And as I came to know myself in this way and meet myself with acceptance and compassion, new ways of being emerged. I discovered alternative pathways to cope with discomfort, to move through transitions, and to honor my grief and longing. It wasn't pretty. There was resistance and rage and so many tears. I suffered bruises and injuries from the battle going on within me—between the part of me that wanted to hold on and the part of me that longed to let go. Those two aspects of me are alive and at work to this day. But grace has taught me to trust the space in between who I was and who I am becoming. And it is there that I experience healing.

I have come to learn that true healing is a whole system that understands our interdependence with everything and everyone around us. Therefore, it acknowledges how we are impacted by the social and environmental conditions that inform our ability to thrive. It also includes the inherited experience of our ancestors and the unknown future state of our descendants. And it never discriminates. It recognizes the lie of normativity as just one more way the system conspires to pull us apart. Healing is about letting go of what is familiar and taking the leap with no guarantee of safety. It holds the contradictions of our human experience—that we are both an ever-evolving work in progress *and* that we are already whole. And it acknowledges that healing looks different to everyone.

PERSONAL INQUIRY

My body answers a gentle call. I lay myself down, cradled by bolsters and blankets, until I am able to soften and surrender. I remember that I am held, despite my pain. My body welcomes me like an old friend. I enter curious and compassionate. It is wild inside of me, full of trapdoors and hidden treasures. I pick up the pieces as I go, gathering all the lost parts of me—the shamed, the neglected, the hurt. Whatever arises, I meet it with a tender breath, a loving embrace, and sometimes forgiveness. I realize that I must love myself back to wholeness. And slowly but surely, I put myself back together again.

- What parts of you have been denied, rejected, neglected that need to be reclaimed?
- What within you needs to be healed and reconciled?
- How do you work with discomfort?
- How have you bought into the idea of "normal"?
- What is your relationship to ableism?
- What does healthy "feel" like to you?

Returning to Wholeness through Healing Justice

One of the things my pain has taught me about my body is how receptive it is to the distress and dysfunction of the outside world. Whenever there is collective chaos, suffering, or injustice, I inevitably feel it through my pain. A "flare-up" is never isolated and always a sensory (often debilitating) response to what is happening around me. It is an invitation to listen to not just what is happening inside me but what is happening in the world. And it is visceral evidence that my self-care is connected to our collective care.

There is no such thing as a single, separate body. Rather, we are an interdependent and unified expression of the whole, complete with impulse and wisdom, heartbreak and hope, joy and pain. It is a collective body that holds within it the history of our suffering and survival and our capacity for resilience and healing. It acknowledges that everything we want to change exists within us and everything that exists within us is shaped by what's around us. If we want to heal, we must acknowledge the systems we are a part of are also sick.

Western medicine has long ignored the mind-body connection, breaking us into separate parts and symptoms to be poked, prodded, and perfected. It asks us to choose between parts of ourselves, trade out dignity for cure, disregard feelings and sensations that don't fit into diagnoses, and strive for someone else's idea of normal and healthy. And it often leaves us feeling more fragmented, scared, and guilty than when it found us. True healing can never be reductionist (the idea that correcting the part will enhance the wholeness). Reductionist approaches to care not only assume that treating a symptom can treat the whole person, they also ignore critical factors that shape our bodies and determine our ability to thrive, including income, housing, education, and access to natural food and water. There is no doubt that modern medicine has given us great, life-saving discoveries and continues to do so. But we can hold that truth while also acknowledging the harm done by the hands of the healers themselves. Our ability to understand how the system works—who's in charge, who's harmed, who benefits, who's excluded—determines how we navigate our way through our suffering and toward the healing we are yearning for.

The medical-industrial complex only works when we believe that if we're sick or suffering it's our fault; that it's not society that's sick, it's *you*. Failure to achieve optimal health (as defined by someone else) results in stigma and shaming that only reinforces our feelings of failure and brokenness. The culture of health as a moral imperative and personal responsibility is the very thing in the way of our healing. Returning to wholeness invites us to locate the problem of injustice and unwellness not in individual bodies and minds but in the world.*

---

* The Healing Histories Project is creating an interactive history of the US medical-industrial complex to expose how "from the beginnings of the institution of colonization and slavery, the state has systematically determined who is 'normal,' 'healthy,' 'diseased,' and 'dangerous' as a way of determining access to its rights and benefits." Understanding our history is essential to healing it and shaping a future of collective care. https://healinghistoriesproject.com.

The mainstream culture of healing has always been rooted in ableism. It focuses on what's wrong with us rather than what's real, natural, and authentic about us. It says that we are either normal or abnormal, fixed or broken, healthy or defective.[32] And it indoctrinates us into a mindset that judges and rejects "defects" while striving for the more perfect and unrealistic version of human potential. According to Mia Mingus, "Ableism is connected to all of our struggles because it undergirds notions of whose bodies are considered valuable, desirable and disposable."[33] Healing in the face of ableism is acknowledging the lies we have bought into. It is directly challenging systems that favor able bodies and oppress everyone else. It is detoxing our mind from the ideologies of healthism and cure that have held us back from our whole selves and our whole communities. And it is creating the conditions where everyone can heal on their terms.

Healing is not one-size-fits-all. Recovering from a dominant system that controls bodies and minds through diagnosis, treatment, and cure means embracing a culture of well-being that is self-determined. When we understand well-being in this way, we can cocreate a system of care and response that conspires to restore us to wholeness. And it's not just about access. It's about agency. Healing is self-determination; it is people deciding for themselves what it means to be well. It's listening and trusting that people know what they need to thrive. And it is uplifting and celebrating the many different expressions that are emerging from the margins, and following their lead. Self-determination is sovereignty—the authority to exert control in our lives, to direct our services, and to act on our own behalf. It is a patient-centered approach to healing that redistributes power and choice from the system to the people.

But self-determination cannot be separated from social justice, in the same way that personal choice cannot be separated from the social determinants of health. True healing demands a complex approach that challenges systems of control and fights for patient access and agency. It speaks to the delicate balance between ancestral healing strategies and our very real reliance on a healthcare system that weaponizes disease and has harmed so many of our communities. Thus, when imagining what a new culture of health and well-being can look like, we should look to the people who have been most marginalized by the current system. The COVID-19 crisis created social, medical, and political trauma that revealed our interdependence—an orientation that has been deeply understood by disabled communities. They have long articulated where and how folks are vulnerable in unjust systems and fought for the very policies that became commonplace during the pandemic. Disability justice emerged to recognize the intersecting legacies of white supremacy, colonialism, capitalism, gendered oppression, and ableism in understanding how people's bodies and minds are labeled "deviant," "unproductive," "disposable," and "invalid." This framework has the power to change the way we think about social change because it demands that we bring our bodies (all of our bodies) back into the conversation and affirms that all bodies are unique and essential.*

Which brings me to healing justice. The concept of healing justice comes out of the work of queer and trans Black, Indigenous, and people of color and was developed by Cara Page and the Atlanta-based Kindred Southern Healing Justice Collective in 2007.[34] It refers to the idea that the systems we seek to change outside of our bodies are also carried within our bodies. It acknowledges that Western systems of care are not innocent; they are rooted in systems of dominance and oppression. It centers the wisdom and leadership of disabled and chronically ill communities who already know about surviving the medical-industrial complex and are reimagining healing for all bodies.† And it remembers that we all come from ancestral medicine and rituals that have been forgotten, erased, stolen, and repackaged by Western culture.

---

* "Nothing about us without us" is a core principle of the disability movement that speaks to how no policies or strategies should be developed without the full and direct participation of those who are most impacted. Follow the lead of Disability Justice organizers like Mia Mingus, Eli Clare, Patty Berne, Leah Lakshmi Piepzna-Samarasinha, Lydia X. Z. Brown, and Sins Invalid.

† One of the podcasts that got me through COVID is *Fortification Podcast COVID-19 Edition*, a powerful series featuring Cara Page, Susan Raffo, and Anjali Taneja and guests about the histories that led to this moment, as well as the present-time expression and future visions needed to transform and intervene on the medical-industrial complex: https://auburnseminary.org/fortification/.

The organizers of the healing justice space at the 2018 Allied Media Conference put it best: "Healing justice is the practice of reimagining wholeness at the intersection of intergenerational trauma, current structures of oppression, and a generative and co-created future. We hold that joy and pleasure create the possibility to be in right relationship with ourselves, each other, and the land. We strive to demystify medicine and healing, and to make them accessible to everyone. We believe that each person is an expert of their own experience, body and needs, and that it is necessary to address the roots of trauma and injustice for individual and collective transformation."[35] Healing justice affirms that personal healing and politicized healing are not separate; they are intertwined practices and strategies intended to disrupt violence, care for communities, and create the conditions for deep and historical healing.*

Recognizing ourselves as both whole and a part of the whole is essential to living in integrity. *Integrity* comes from the word *integer*, which means "to become whole and complete." The practice of integrity is remembering that we already are. Healing doesn't require that we return to "normal" or the "before" state. Healing is the full inclusion and integration of our bodies and lived experiences, so that we can move through the world whole. It is how we love each other and let each other be. Healing is who we are beyond our wounds and because of them. It is how we let the old parts of us die to allow for new growth. It is the most terrible and the most beautiful thing that has ever happened to us. It is ours and it is up to us. Author Cheryl Strayed reminds us that "when you recognize that you will thrive not in spite of your losses and sorrows, but because of them . . . the word for that is *healing*."[36]

---

* To learn more about healing justice, check out the Kindred Southern Healing Justice Collective, Transform Harm, the Embody Institute, BEAM, and Just Practice, and follow healing justice leaders Cara Page, Shira Hassan, Susan Raffo, Prentis Hemphill, and Yolo Akili.

COLLECTIVE PRACTICE: CENTER IN WHOLENESS

Healing is a constant practice of coming back to ourselves over and over and over again. When we can learn to tolerate our own aliveness—feelings, fears, experiences, emotions—we can show up more fully for our collective healing. Centering meditation is an embodied practice that calls us to embrace our whole selves in relationship to everything and everyone around us. It invites us to become fully present to whatever we are experiencing and explore our full capacity to meet each moment and respond to what is needed. From center we can both heal backward and generate forward.

- Find a position where your body feels supported and spacious to the extent that it makes sense in your body (it can be seated, standing, supine, or something else).* Connect to a steady breath and lower your gaze.† Listen to what's going on in your body. You might notice sensation or activation or even dullness. See if you can allow whatever is coming up.

- Bring your attention to your roots—whatever part of your body feels grounded and connected to the earth or support system beneath you. Your roots are both firm and yielding, generous and reciprocal. Notice how you are held by the earth—supported and resourced in every moment. Let it affirm your connection with the earth, that you are not just on it but of it.

---

* Centering can be done in any body. I did my best to make this embodied exercise accessible to different bodies, but I acknowledge that my perspective is limited and there may be things that don't make sense for you. Listen to your body and adapt as necessary.

† If connecting to breath doesn't feel supportive, bring your attention to a place in the body that feels grounding.

- From deep roots, draw upward through the legs, feeling the kneecaps and thighs lift. Continue to harness the energy through the core of the body, climbing up through the spine and lengthening out through the crown of the head. Feel yourself embody dignity. My favorite definition of dignity is "knowing that your best is good enough." What does it feel like to know and carry that in your body? That your best is good enough?

- Keeping that vertical line that is both rooting and rising, now breathe into the back side of the body. This part of the body represents everything that came before this moment. It is the places we have been, the experiences we have gone through, the people who have crossed our paths. But it is also those who came before, our ancestors who did the best they could so that we could be here in this way today. Lean back into the wisdom and the knowledge that is at your back and in your bones.

- Now open the front of your body to all that is in front of you. It is uncertain and out of our control. Can you open your heart with faith to the future that we belong to?

- Take a breath now into your width, allowing the waist and ribs to expand. It is through this part of the body that we understand that we are not alone. Expand your breath, and see if you can include the people around you and all who are with you on this path. Let yourself take up space, and trust that there is enough room for everyone to express and expand into their full potential.

- Finally, feel into every direction—how we root to rise, how we lean back into the wisdom we come from to open to the future we are becoming, how we expand in relationship to include and embrace all living things—and connect to the whole of who you are, the you that is already whole. It is from this place that we remember who we are and can heal forward.

Healing the whole of who we are demands that we go back and recover the parts of ourselves that we've left behind. And I don't just mean our personal selves, because there is no individual healing that is separate from the healing of the whole. True healing and well-being are only possible when we actively engage in the healing of our communities, our systems, our culture, and our history.

CHAPTER 3

The Myth of Wellness

Shouting self-care at people who actually need community care is how we fail people.

NIKITA VALERIO

When I found yoga, everything changed. Instead of fixing and controlling, I started to let myself feel. The yoga mat was more like a wrestling mat—the place where I faced my pain and my fear and my loss. And it was messy. But something was happening and the more I moved and breathed through it, the more my grief changed. The practice wasn't just healing me, it was revealing me, this new version of me, so much so that I quit my job, moved across the country, became a yoga teacher, and vowed to change the world.

I arrived in San Francisco in 2002, just as wellness was taking off. On any given day, you would either find me at the yoga studio, the Whole Foods, or the Lululemon. I was as woo-woo as they come: adorned in mala beads and $100 yoga pants with my tried-and-true yoga mat slung across my back. I would lecture my friends and family on the benefits of meditation and recite sutras to anyone who would listen. I felt like I was a part of something magical—people were waking up, eating organic, buying green everything, piling into yoga studios like it was Coachella. We were hungry for meaning and hope and connection, and I was obsessed . . . I would hit my mat, stalk organic food, and seek exotic retreats like my life depended on it.

The post-yoga glow was real. I would emerge from savasana cleansed in sweat and liberated from whatever weight and worry I had carried onto my mat. There are lots of words used to describe that feeling—bliss, ecstasy, contentment—when you come back to yourself and know it is going to be OK, when you feel hopeful again. I would savor that glow in the sanctuary of my studio for as long as I could. And then I would blissfully step out onto Folsom and Fourth with my green juice in hand and walk right into the same group of homeless youth who took shelter in that stoop every evening. Clad in piercings and punk gear, they were inconspicuous in how they blended into their surroundings. And yet they demanded to be seen. At first I would plow by, too busy to notice. Then I started to look. Eventually I just stopped, unable to ignore what was right there in front of me.

The world outside of my wellness bubble was different. Really different. From domestic violence to ongoing wars, from chronic illness to medical trauma, from starving children to food apartheid—people were struggling to survive, much less be well.

I realized that my yoga practice wasn't just revealing me, it was revealing the real world in living color. And no matter how much I tried to meditate it away, I couldn't unsee the suffering all around me. I used to think it was enough to have good intentions, to be a healthy and compassionate citizen. But then I wondered if that was just a myth that enabled me to escape. And I began to grapple with why I got to be well when others didn't. How well-being had somehow become a privilege afforded to people with access and time and money. People like me.

We've Been Goop'd

Against the backdrop of a booming tech industry and homelessness crisis, San Francisco was a budding mecca of wellness, filled with fog and hippies and really fucking healthy people. Patchouli-incensed yoga studios, crowded vegan restaurants, Himalayan boutiques filled with prayer flags and Ganesh statues, the Bay was a weird and totally wonderful counterculture. In the twenty years that have passed since I first arrived in San Francisco, wellness has gone mainstream, the landscape crowded with aspiring images and alluring ads inviting you into the next best version of yourself. From juice bars and meditation retreats to crystals and mindfulness apps, these trending health fads show no sign of abating. Wellness is hip-hop yoga. It's a rose quartz face roller. It's vegan and paleo and macrobiotic. Wellness is yoga mats at Walmart and clean beauty at Target. It's collagen supplements, vitamin B shots, and elixirs. It's Beyond Burgers at Burger King. It's skin glow gummies and mushroom adaptogens. It's hot springs, silent retreats, essential oils. Wellness is manifesting mantras and charging one's chakras. It's juice fasts, gluten-free, and oat milk. Wellness is in school, at work, on vacation, in the airport. Wellness is everywhere.

To understand how we got here, we must go back. While wellness has manifestations in the nineteenth century (especially among aristocrats with the time and money to explore new thought, health trends, and alternative medicine), it wasn't really established until the 1950s, when Dr. Halbert Dunn drew a distinction between good health as a passive state of not being ill and what he termed "high-level wellness," or "a condition of change in which the individual moves forward, climbing toward a higher potential of functioning."[1] It made prime time in 1979 when Dan Rather ran a segment on *60 Minutes*, opening with, "Wellness, that's not a word you hear every day."[2] Cut to today, and the wellness mindset has permeated all aspects of our lives. And wellness wouldn't be where it's at without the phenomenon of yoga.

The origins of the ancient practice of yoga go back many thousands of years, but the modern roots can be traced to 1893, when East met West at the Parliament of the World's Religions. Swami Vivekananda, a Hindu Indian monk, traveled to Chicago and gave a brief talk on September 11, 1893. His speech, which spoke of universal tolerance and compassion for the persecuted, boldly challenged Western ideas of imperialism and presented a spiritual unity that transcends religion; it made him an instant sensation.[3] But while Vivekananda's daring political ideas may have opened the door for yoga in America, the culture of yoga that hooked me and millions of others did not come from his legacy, but from an unassuming white woman from eastern Europe.

Indra Devi, born Eugenia Peterson at the turn of the century in the Russian Empire (today's Latvia), came of age during the New Thought movement (an ancestor to New Age). An aspiring actress and spiritual seeker, she traveled to India and became the first female student of Tirumalai Krishnamacharya, often referred to as the father of modern yoga.[4] Krishnamacharya created the posture-based yoga practice that we know today, a physical system of yoga that pulled from mystical yogic tradition, Indian wrestling practices, British army calisthenics, martial arts, and more. Devi was able to bring yoga west when many South Asians could not because of the Immigration Act of 1924, which barred immigration from Asia and set quotas and restrictions on immigration from other "less desirable" countries in eastern and southern Europe.[5] Her dress style (white woman clad in saris) immediately attracted a following of movie stars and Hollywood housewives eager for the "exotic" practices of the East that promised to keep them forever young and beautiful. And that is the story of how a white woman brought yoga west and seeded what would become the modern wellness movement.*

In the twenty-first century, wellness has reached a dramatic tipping point. Valued at over $4.3 trillion worldwide, according to the Global Wellness Institute, wellness far surpasses the pharmaceutical market ($1 trillion).[6] The industry has been growing at a rate of 6.4 percent per year, and it has successfully permeated the consciousness of the consumer, affecting everyday decision-making such as healthy food purchases, mindfulness for stress reduction, essential oils for wrinkles, mind-body fitness, and eco-friendly products.[7] No longer a niche, wellness for many people in the US and around the world has evolved from the occasional to the essential, from luxury to lifestyle.

---

* In *Goddess Pose*, Michelle Goldberg tells the provocative story of Indra Devi and how yoga came west.

And it's no wonder people are turning to wellness. Modern medicine has failed to curb the growing epidemic of noncommunicable and preventable diseases such as heart attacks, diabetes, and chronic illness, which have become the US's leading killers.[8] The medical-industrial complex isn't motivated by making people well, it's motivated by making money. Add to that an unhealthy and unregulated food system deeply entrenched by money in politics and the human-made harm to our environment that threatens extinction, it's not surprising that people seek out an alternative system that promises to make us better. All of which has inspired an aggressive culture of kale-eating, crystal-loving consumers who can't get enough.

And I was one of them, desperate and hungry for healing. The wellness industry promised to make me feel good, look better, get healthy, and become a more attractive version of myself. Wellness wasn't just some hobby; it was an ambitious pursuit of something better. I became obsessed with perfecting poses, eating right, sounding enlightened, and being seen. Belonging to the wellness world demanded that I play the part, aspire for enlightenment, and strive to become my best self as prescribed by Goop.

What began as a sort of voyeurism of Gwyneth Paltrow living her best life has become a $250 million lifestyle brand that is making a killing off of women who want what Gwyneth has. It has spawned a website, a magazine, a podcast, a Netflix series, and myriad products from creams to crystals to vibrators. Goop has become a one-stop shop for individuals obsessed with what Gwyneth calls the "optimization of the self." "We're here one time, one life, like how can we really, like, milk the shit out of this," she says.[9] By milking it she means a $495 vibrator and a $295 incense holder and a $350 meditation headband. Who can afford that? I certainly couldn't. But I would try.

You see, woven between seemingly feminist messages of empowerment and healing is an insidious wellness culture exploiting our insecurities, propping up healthism, and getting rich along the way. Everywhere we turn, it tells us we're not good enough. It says, "Buy this and you will be happy, do this and you will feel beautiful, eat this and you will be healthy, read this and you will be enlightened." It is a storyline sponsored by a system that profits from our sickness.

And like 80 million other Americans, I believed it. I bought it. I even sold it.

The Well-Being Gap

What I couldn't see in my yoga stupor is that while the wellness economy soars, so does inequality. Inequality has been a staple of the so-called American Dream for as long as we've had one. It's why the US is both the wealthiest and the most unequal country among industrialized nations. While one part of the country is making choices about organic and GMO-free food, the rest of the country is trying to figure out how to pay their bills and feed their families. The irony of wellness is that behind its promise of unity is a deep divide.

The well-being gap is the unequal conditions that determine who gets to be well and who doesn't. It is the gap of all gaps. It is an intersectional lens that considers the many interlocking (and imbalanced) systems that impact our ability to be well. It is the health gap where rates of preventable chronic diseases, which account for 70 percent of deaths in the US, disproportionately impact low-income communities; it is the maternal mortality gap that affects Black women at 3.3 times and Indigenous women at 2.5 times the rate of white women; it is the wealth gap where the richest 10 percent has 70 percent of total household wealth in America; it is the justice gap that incarcerates Black boys at 4 times the rate of white boys.[10] But perhaps the best indicator of the well-being gap is life expectancy—how the richest Americans live ten to fifteen years longer than the poorest Americans. And according to the Health Inequality Project, that gap is only getting wider.[11]

A well-being gap that leaves *some* people behind hurts all of us. It destabilizes our economy, causes stress that makes us sick, fuels higher rates of crime and violence, holds back our children, and separates us from each other. And here's the kicker . . . the cost of that gap in America is upward of $500 billion.[12] These are not someone else's problems. These are our problems, all of us. And while it may be easy for some of us to turn away and

72

stay in our gated communities of wellness, we must instead turn toward the hard-to-look-at truth of our people and planet.

But I didn't want to "look" at the truth of our suffering. I wanted to stay in the comfort and ignorance of my yoga bubble. I wanted to be right about wellness—that we could be saved by meditation and mantras. But I was in for a rude awakening. No amount of green juice and yoga poses is going to get us well as long as many people around us are suffering. And while it is tempting to try to find ourselves through personal practice and a healthy lifestyle, in happiness apps and expensive supplements, we only become more lost and isolated. When we tie our well-being to something that can be purchased or achieved outside of ourselves, it hooks us in a never-ending cycle of accumulation that only further perpetuates the gap.

But that is not what we are being sold. The ideology of wellness culture is one of personal responsibility, isolated acts, and moral codes. In *The Wellness Syndrome*, Carl Cederström and André Spicer describe it as "infectious narcissism" that assumes that if we all just took better care of ourselves and were a little more positive, all would be right in the world.[13] But the trade-offs are real. "The unemployed are not provided with an income; they get life coaching. Discriminated groups don't get opportunities to celebrate their identities, they get an exercise plan. Citizens don't get the opportunity to influence decisions that affect their lives; they get a mindfulness session. Meanwhile, inequality, discrimination and authoritarianism become seen as questions too grand to tackle head on. Instead, political ambitions become myopically focused on boosting our well-being."[14]

This culture betrays us in the following ways: First it convinces us that if we are sick, sad, and exhausted, that's our fault. It's not the economy or structural imbalances or systemic injustice, it's you. "The lexis of abuse and gaslighting is appropriate here," says journalist and screenwriter Laurie Penny. "If you are miserable or angry because your life is a constant struggle against privation or prejudice, the problem is always and only with you. Society is not mad or messed up. You are."[15] The other thing it does is try to sell us individual solutions to what it tells us are individual problems (which they're not). Stressed out because you are juggling two jobs and raising kids? You should try meditation. Feeling powerless and depressed because you are out of work? There is a mantra for that. Suffering from the symptoms of your chronic disease? Gluten-free can fix that. Can't afford to go to yoga? Manifest abundance.

And yet, despite all these well-marketed wellness solutions, chronic disease, which accounts for 70 percent of deaths in the US, is on the rise.[16] When wellness culture masks or neglects the systemic barriers that are in the way of being well, it prevents us from engaging in an appropriate collective response to the very real crises of unemployment, poverty, lack of access to healthy food and healthcare, and more. As community activist Chloe Ann-King puts it, "Changing your attitude is not going to change or help dismantle structural injustice and a failed and unsustainable economic model, which serves only the elite rich in this world and exploits the rest of us."[17] Positive thinking and magical manifestation are particularly bitter pills to swallow in the context of rampant inequality.

The personal-choices myth has resulted in widespread stereotypes that poor people are sick because they are smoking, drinking, and eating fast food, despite the fact that lifestyle is not a primary driver of life expectancy.[18] What is responsible for a majority of this gap is poverty itself. All humans experience stress, but the experience of chronic stress is not evenly distributed across society. Research shows that people are more likely to experience stress-related diseases (e.g., heart disease, diabetes, asthma, and anxiety) when they lack adequate support and control over dealing with stressful conditions.[19] Those who are poor disproportionately face such conditions. But poverty never works in isolation. It is intertwined with other sites of oppression like racism, ableism, and sexism.

That's why "equality" is not enough. Equality assumes that everyone is starting from the same place. It involves treating everyone in a similar manner despite their differences or needs. Equality is about sameness. Equity on the other hand acknowledges that, because of our history of oppression and the structural injustices people are born into, we are not all starting from the same place and, therefore, have different needs to survive and thrive. It is not enough to frame this as disparity without acknowledging that these health *differences* are actually health *inequities*—that they are not only avoidable and preventable, they are also unfair and unjust, rooted in social injustices that make some groups more vulnerable to poor health than other groups. This analysis is critical in determining how to bridge the gap. The concept of equality denies people their experience of being excluded, under-resourced, invalidated, and exploited; its insistence on responding to difference with sameness will also prevent us from ever getting where we need to go.*

The Violence of Inequality

I wrote this book in 2020 and early 2021, as COVID-19 swept the country. Highly infectious respiratory diseases like COVID-19 pose a threat to everyone in society. But while viruses don't discriminate, inequities do, revealing the very unequal conditions that determine who gets to live and who doesn't. The coronavirus didn't expose me to contagion as much as it exposed my privilege: how being a relatively able-bodied, immuno-healthy entrepreneur who gets to work from home inoculated me from becoming infected with the virus. As hospital beds filled up and the death toll rose, I continued to thrive in superior health, fortified by my immune supplements—and on the backs of essential workers. That's right, no part of my survival would have been possible were it not for the farmhands and grocery store workers who kept me well fed, or the delivery drivers who made it possible for me to stay at home, or the invisible engineers who maintained the grid and kept my beloved internet going. Essential workers took risks so that people like me could thrive.

The decisions of who gets a test, who gets to use the ventilator, who gets to work from home, and who gets to be well are inescapably shaped by inequity. Those who are most vulnerable—people who are elderly, poor, disabled, immunocompromised, undocumented, houseless, and essential workers—are least proximal to the access and resources needed to survive. For everyone else, self-quarantines and social distancing reveal the reality

---

* There is a thoughtful exploration of equity vs. equality in the blog post "The Problem with That Equity vs. Equality Graphic You're Using" by Paul Kuttner: http://www.socialventurepartners .org/wp-content/uploads/2018/01/Problem-with-Equity-vs-Equality-Graphic.pdf.

of isolation that undocumented, disabled, and elderly folks have been living for a very long time. A pandemic can teach us everything we need to know about public health. It brings into sharper view what has been there all along: that wellness is a privilege for those who have access, time, and money. Equality is not possible in a system that is set up to privilege some and oppress others. And no amount of positive thinking or elderberry is going to fix that.

Issues of poverty, housing, access to healthcare, and employment are much more likely to inform one's health than personal choice is. Social determinants of health (unlike the biomedical model, which solely focuses on the individual) address the unequal allocation of goods (e.g., access to healthy food), services (e.g., access to healthcare), and attention (e.g., responsiveness of systems of care), which manifest in unequal and unhealthy social, economic, and environmental conditions.* Even smoking, which is associated with more diseases than any other behavior, doesn't happen in isolation; it is a product of social interaction and smoking-prone environments. Like fish in a fishbowl, the health and well-being of human beings are deeply affected by the conditions in which we live, learn, work, play, worship, and grow old.

Take Tribeca, for example, a predominantly white community in Manhattan that enjoys wealth, high income, "good schools," and low crime. Residents have an average life expectancy of eighty-five years of age. Less than eight miles away in Brownsville, Brooklyn, the average life expectancy is only seventy-four.[20] What's the difference? Ninety-six percent of Brownville residents are people of color, 40 percent live in poverty, which is twice the poverty rate of the city as a whole, and more than half of Brownsville's children live in poverty, far above the city's child poverty rate of 30 percent.[21] This trend envelops our nation, where people of color, particularly Black and Indigenous communities, are disproportionately impacted by poverty compared to the rest of the population and face higher rates of preventable

---

* *The Health Gap: The Challenge of an Unequal World* by Michael Marmot looks at the relationship between inequality and health disparities on a global scale.

chronic diseases such as diabetes, asthma, stroke, and heart disease. The health disparities for Indigenous people are the worst among all racial groups, resulting in lower life expectancy, lower quality of life, and a higher prevalence of many chronic conditions. When you start to really look at where the sickness is, you find it is not what's in the individual as much as it is what's around the individual.

Place-based health inequities don't just happen by accident. They stem from a historical strategy to designate which neighborhoods are worthy of investment and allocation of resources. For example, redlining—the practice of discriminating against residents of an area based on their race or ethnicity through systematic policies that discourage loans and investments—originated during the Great Depression when red lines were drawn on maps around neighborhoods whose residents were predominantly Black, segregating them in areas that were significantly under-resourced in basic infrastructure development and overexposed to environmental threats. These practices have effectively shaped many of the demographic and wealth patterns of American communities. And while redlining is no longer legal, its legacy correlates directly to some of the biggest economic and health gaps between people of color and white people today.*

Structural inequity begins at the womb. Black infants die at twice the rate of white infants; the disparity is even more acute in busy urban areas like San Francisco, where Black mothers are twice as likely to lose their babies as white mothers.[22] Add to that the fact that Black women are 3.2 times more likely to die from complications of pregnancy than white women.[23] What our maternal and infant mortality rates are telling us is that the gap between who gets to survive and who doesn't goes way beyond the social determinants of health. Black women and their families report disparities in access and care. Not only are their symptoms often dismissed, but 25 percent report disrespect and abuse by medical professionals.[24] And while the medical-industrial complex often attributes preexisting conditions among Black women as the

---

* For more on the history of redlining, check out *Race for Profit: How Banks and the Real Estate Industry Undermined Black Homeownership* by Keeanga-Yamahtta Taylor.

reason for the disproportionate maternal mortality rate and other health disparities, the data points to racial discrimination (rather than race itself) as the reason so many Black women and babies are dying in childbirth.* Preexisting conditions are not the comorbidity. Structural racism is.[25]

When examining the root causes of inequity, it's not enough to address the social determinants of health. We must also acknowledge the systemic mechanisms that deliberately organize and distribute resources across lines of race, gender, class, sexual orientation, and other dimensions of individual and group identity. Connected to that are power structures that control who gets taken care of and who doesn't. The term *structural violence* goes further by acknowledging the structures *that are designed* to keep in place the inequities that viciously determine who gets to be well and who doesn't. In *Pathologies of Power: Health, Human Rights, and the New War on the Poor* author and medical anthropologist Paul Farmer says, "The most basic right—the right to survive—is trampled in an age of great affluence, and . . . should be considered the most pressing one of our times."[26] The coronavirus pandemic bluntly exposed the structural violence that caused Black, Indigenous, Latinx, and Asian American people to be infected at disproportionate rates. The ecosystem was ripe for this, already codified by racist legislation and structures that resulted in poverty, subpar housing, environmental racism, preexisting health conditions, and unequal access to healthcare, all of which make people more vulnerable to the disease. People were already dying a slow death in this structure before the pandemic hit. It was just invisible to those who didn't want to see it.[†]

---

* Black Mamas Matter Alliance is a Black-women-led cross-sectoral alliance that centers Black mamas to advocate, drive research, build power, and shift culture for Black maternal health, rights, and justice. Check out their toolkit to advance Black maternal health: http://blackmamasmatter.org/wp-content/uploads/2018/05/USPA_BMMA_Toolkit_Booklet-Final-Update_Web-Pages-1.pdf.

† In *Inflamed: Deep Medicine and the Anatomy of Injustice*, Rupa Marya and Raj Patel reveal the hidden relationships between our biological systems and the profound injustices of our political and economic systems.

The Privilege of Wellness

Wellness culture is deeply out of touch. The single mother working two full-time, low-wage jobs is unlikely to get adequate sleep, much less make time for a daily yoga class or meditation practice. The disabled elder whose only income is a tiny social security check may not be able to access a health food store, much less afford the organic produce there. The young person living in an urban, densely packed housing project near the industrial side of town may have a hard time exercising when the air isn't safe to breathe. The privilege of wellness has been right there in front of us all along.

Privilege simply means you have a leg up, an advantage. There are many sites of privilege that shape our experience in America and inform how we move in the world. Simply being born in this country affords a person certain privileges a noncitizen will never access. Growing up in a family that is financially stable affects your health, safety, education, and opportunities. Straight people are automatically guaranteed spousal benefits in every state that gay, lesbian, bisexual, and queer people have had to fight for. Most men can walk through a dark alley without worrying they will be raped (and face a defense attorney who will blame it on what they were wearing). If you are cisgender, you likely don't worry that the restroom or locker room you use will invoke harassment or violence. If you aren't disabled, you don't have to fear that everything from basic daily activities to life-saving care might be denied to you due to lack of necessary accommodations or assumptions about the value of your life and your ability to self-determine. And none of these identities acts in isolation. Being born into one or more categories of privilege "can be like winning a lottery you didn't even know you were playing," as Gina Crosley-Corcoran puts it.[27]

I won that lottery. My privileged identities are too many to count: white, cis, nondisabled, middle-class, educated, natural-born citizen. But it's not just who I am, it's how I have benefited. It is the privilege of growing up in a white, middle-class, "safe" neighborhood with "good" schools. It is the advantage of ableism that meant that for most of my life I never had to think about how to enter a building or whether there would be seating for my body. It is the privilege of feeling like it's possible to "not see color" and wishing we could all just get along. It is how law enforcement gives me the benefit of the doubt. It is having endless choices about where to live and what to do in the world. This is where I would typically shut down in guilt and shame. But I know better now—that is just one more way the system works to silence us. Privilege must be realized, so that we can work with it and not around it.

Having privilege doesn't mean that your life is easy; it means that one or more aspects of who you are don't make it harder. Society is designed to meet the needs of those with privilege in ways that are invisible to us and yet expected. It's how people like me, who come from more privileged populations, are more likely to have our everyday food items stocked at the supermarket. Or how we are more likely to see ourselves reflected in TV shows and the media. Or how we are more likely to be given the benefit of the doubt when seeking a financial loan. And to be clear, privilege is absolutely tied to the ability to accumulate wealth and security in this country. For example, the racial wealth gap remains as wide in 2020 as it was in 1968, with the net worth of a typical white family being nearly ten times greater than that of a black family.[28] People with disabilities earn 34 percent less total income than nondisabled individuals.[29] Trans and nonbinary people experience poverty at four times the national average.[30] And history matters in contemporary inequality, where privilege is passed down from generation to generation, further entrenching the well-being gap.

But privilege is not neutral. It is part of larger power structures that determine who gets to be well and who doesn't. Well-being is situated in those power structures, creating the terms that determine who gets access, who feels safe, who gets to lead. But privilege is also how we use spirituality to avoid the harsh reality of our world and explain away people's lived experiences. Phrases like "everything happens for a reason" and "positive vibes only" are code for "your suffering and sickness is your fault, and only you can change it." It upholds privilege by dismissing the very real and justified lived experiences of people who are oppressed and absolves people of privilege of their responsibility to be accountable and confront injustice. Spiritual bypass is an opt-out for those who can afford to look the other way.* And while it may uphold the status quo, it isn't going to get you well.

The irony is that true well-being demands that we turn toward the truth and discomfort of our experience in order to transform it. Well-being understands that justice is needed to bring systems of privilege and oppression into balance. It reveals our connection to all things and the fact that none of us can truly be well unless everyone is well. There is no well-being that avoids, neglects, erases, and excludes. If we want to be well, we're going to need to embrace our discomfort, confront our privilege, and fight for the conditions where everyone can thrive.

---

* John Welwood coined the term "spiritual bypass," and Robert Augustus Masters wrote the seminal book on the subject: *Spiritual Bypass: When Spirituality Disconnects Us from What Really Matters.*

RECOVERY

You cannot change any society unless you take responsibility for it, unless you see yourself belonging to it and
responsible for changing it.

GRACE LEE BOGGS

Looking back, I wonder if what drew me to wellness was not so much the desire to be well but the desire to be purified. The world is a toxic mess full of suffering and violence and injustice, and I didn't just want to escape—I wanted to transcend it. The promise of purity and the seduction of hope gave me a way out, a bypass to the discomfort of both my suffering and my privilege. Wellness promised to make me better, to absolve me of my toxic ways and deliver me anew. These self-righteous protocols to eat clean, to avoid inflammation, to think positive thoughts imply that we can rise above it all. But there is no such thing as purity in a world polluted by separation, scarcity, and supremacy.

Thus began my reckoning with wellness. On one hand, I had discovered in wellness a way of being and belonging that felt true and right on so many levels. On the other hand, that very culture was reinforcing the very illness and imbalance it was intended to address. I felt betrayed by the very thing that had offered me refuge and healing when I needed it most, leaving me only more isolated and unwell. No longer could I reconcile my personal pursuit of wellness with the suffering that was all around me.

Inevitably (and ironically) I discovered the truth on my mat. I was hips-deep in a yoga class in San Francisco, moving through confusion and sweating through my discomfort. Our teacher, Seane Corn, was leading us in an excruciating flow that alternated between passionate instruction and prophetic inquiry. Her classes were like a rite of passage—an invitation to confront our demons and connect with our higher self. And in the middle of what seemed like an unethically long pigeon pose, she asked a question that would change my life forever: *"What if you took your yoga off the mat and into the world?"* Those words landed so fully in my body. And I realized that yoga and wellness weren't about feeling good or escaping the truth, they were about turning toward the truth and asking "How can I be of service?" Soon after, I would end up running an organization of the same name that was committed to bridging personal transformation and social change.

Dissonance is the discomfort one feels when faced with conflicting truths, and it is most painful when it strikes at the heart of how we see ourselves. But when faced with the discomfort of contradiction, we have a choice. We can either dig in and retreat to our individual wellness bubbles or we can lean in and let ourselves be implicated and impacted by our shared humanity. Once I gave in to that, I could no longer unsee the suffering all around me, nor could I bypass my part in that. And here's the best part. Coming to terms with my privilege and my place in this mess was the very thing that revealed my purpose and path forward. I wasn't here to do yoga and be well, I was here to fight for the conditions where everyone gets to thrive on their terms.

The paradox of wellness is one to behold. There's no amount of meditation and yoga that can save us from soaring poverty or record incarceration or the destruction of our planet. Reconciling these two things is going to demand more than increased access and acts of charity. It's going to require a paradigm shift at every level. It begins with our own consciousness about where and how we are privileged in systems of health and well-being and how to respond and act from that place of awareness. It invites us to challenge the spaces and systems that uphold inequities and to advocate for conditions that enable people to feel taken care of and free to express themselves. And it calls us to push back against a wellness culture that justifies the well-being gap as a product of personal choice and not systemic inequities. For well-being to work, it must address fundamental issues of inequity and exclusion; it must imagine new, more inclusive and authentic systems that take care of everyone. Closing the well-being gap is going to take all of us. All of us who believe we can—and need to—do better for ourselves, our communities, and our society.

Reckoning with the Privilege of Wellness

It wasn't until I discovered what yoga isn't that I truly understood what it really is. Yoga is not an escape from the harsh realities of our world. It is not a blissed-out bright-siding of the truth of who we are and where we come from.* And it is not the exclusion of any part of our experience or history. *Yoga* means "to yoke," to unite all the disparate parts of ourselves without exception. It invites us to confront the personal and collective obstacles that are in the way of our liberation. Yoga is rooted in an ancient principle called *ahimsa* in Sanskrit, which means "non-harming," a concept that can be found in South Asia's karmic religions including Hinduism, Buddhism, and Jainism. In other words, any expression of yoga or wellness that contributes to the suffering, exclusion, exploitation, or oppression of others is not yoga at all, it's just more suffering. The real yoga is off the mat. It is how we show up in service and action for the well-being of everyone.

Dominant culture encourages personal responsibility, which allows some of us to insulate and "mind our business," but humanity is saying something very different. We see it in the manifestation of the climate crisis that is triggering natural disasters that don't discriminate. We experience it in contagious disease that exposes the danger of valuing individual liberties over collective well-being. And we feel it in the economic fallout from an enormous gulf in wealth distribution. No matter our level of privilege or insulation, no matter how distant we may feel from those who are directly to blame for such crises, we are mutually responsible for what is being perpetuated by our culture, for what's playing out in our communities, for the systems and the structures that have been created to keep things a certain way. These are not someone else's problems; they are our problems, all of us.†

---

* *Bright-Sided: How the Relentless Promotion of Positive Thinking Has Undermined America* by Barbara Ehrenreich exposes how harmful the "positive thinking" movement is—how it means self-blame, victim blaming, and national denial.

† Mutuality does not mean equality. It understands that the impacts of inequality are landing on and in our bodies in disproportionate ways.

When we rely on individual responses to solve systemic problems, we remain stuck. Underneath wellness culture's feel-good philosophy is that what sells relief from participating in toxic systems, in reality, ends up blaming individuals for our own unhappiness. And the products that companies claim are sustainable and will make us healthier are the very ones causing harm and reinforcing systems of oppression. Consider the sweatshops that are used to produce sexy yoga leggings, or the wellness magazines that reinforce normative bodies, or the demand for superfoods like quinoa that is putting Indigenous farmers out of business. Nothing exemplifies this more than the fact that the US makes up 5 percent of the global population but consumes 25 percent of the world's resources—finite resources that are being rapidly depleted.[31] Not only is this unsustainable, but it implicates all of us who live a privileged lifestyle in America. And yet our impulse is often to respond to complex social issues with the attitude of "it's not my problem." Dominant culture reinforces the belief that if we just meditate, eat organic, and drive a hybrid we are making our contribution to the world. But this individualized view not only keeps us from doing our part, it keeps us from truly being well.

That's not to say there is no role for personal responsibility and the inquiry of "How can I as an individual do the right thing, reduce harm, and support the realignment of resources toward equity?" There is, but it's not the whole of it. We need to locate our personal responsibility inside of mutuality. Understanding our social location—our social group memberships that determine our proximity to power, privilege, and even wellness—is how we skillfully engage in a wellness that takes care of all of us, not just some of us. And seeing ourselves as part of the problem and part of the solution moves us toward one another. Mutual responsibility reminds us that there can be no well-being of me unless there is a well-being of we. Interdependence affirms that there is no separation—that we are all impacted by one another. Mutuality is a generative worldview that grows and expands with equity. Not only is there enough to go around for everyone to be well, but more well-being creates more well-being.

All of this invites us to reckon with our privilege. Most of us are privileged in one or many ways, even if we also experience marginalization in other ways. Privilege isn't your fault, but it is your responsibility. And this is where most people quit. Our need to defend our goodness and innocence overrides any attempt to reckon with the truth of our complicity. But any instinct to retreat or protect your comfort only serves to uphold the systems that created it. Instead, consider taking inventory of your privilege and becoming aware of how the system works to advantage you. You can start by asking "What do I have that I didn't earn?" to help interrogate the advantages we carry around with us that often go unseen. A good follow-up is "Who created that system?" and "What keeps it going?" Because privilege doesn't happen by accident. It's designed that way.

That's because privilege works in collusion with oppression in that it is only possible at the expense of others. It functions to pit one group against another. And while it is easy to focus on oppression of "others"— or even ourselves—and how people have been unjustly denied resources, inclusion, and validation, it's harder to acknowledge one's privilege. Probably because it implicates those who have it. It doesn't matter whether you earned privilege or not; having it makes you a part of a system that benefits from the oppression of others. Privilege and oppression are inseparable. And the data is indisputable, bringing to life the documented health disparities between people with the most privilege and people with the least. But here's the thing of it—a well-being gap that advantages some and disadvantages others isn't making any of us well.

It wasn't enough to wake up to privilege. Healing required that I do something with it—that I try to stop the cycle of harm that my privilege is caught up in. No longer could I experience the serenity of my yoga class without seriously confronting the homeless crisis outside the yoga studio's door. So I took my practice to GLIDE, a landmark center for social justice in San Francisco, and began offering yoga to local residents who dropped in for hot meals and housing. Unlike the spa-like aesthetic of my former studio, this yoga space was grounded by linoleum floors, draped in stacked folding chairs, infused with the aroma of the mess hall downstairs, and adjacent to sounds of the local bus stop. But yoga happened here. And it was the most real yoga I had ever experienced.

Privilege is not only about what we know but what we owe. And while it's not really possible to give away privilege in a culture that is designed around it, you can leverage your proximity to people and systems of privilege to educate, disrupt, challenge, and change. You can look for ways to educate the people around you with whom you share social-group memberships about privilege so that they, too, can become more aware and skilled about how to navigate inequity. And you can risk your privilege to disrupt a system of inequity and benefit others. This looks like intervening when people in power are causing harm. It looks like getting out of the way, so that less-privileged folks can have a greater share of voice and power. It looks like advocating for conditions that people need to not just survive but thrive. It looks like redistributing access, resources, and power to those who have been systematically marginalized and oppressed. And it looks like a willingness to give something up because we believe that a culture that takes care of everyone will get us all free.

Often an awareness of one's privilege prompts calls for diversification. And while diversification is a start, it's not enough. Even the idea that we have to *include* assumes that someone "own[s] the table" as Ruby Sales, human rights activist and public theologian, notes—someone is making the decisions, someone is deciding for us what it means to be well or to be worthy.[32] We don't need more people like me deciding what well-being is, what well-being looks like, making the rules for how well-being should work. It's not enough to want to make unequal systems more inclusive. True well-being is confronting and correcting whatever is in the way of our collective wholeness. It's risking our comfort and doing our part to ensure everyone has what they need to thrive.

I realize now how small and limiting my idea of wellness once was. As if navel-gazing and hoarding wellness could save me. But there is no getting well for any of us in a system designed to reinforce inequity and pit us against each other. True wellness is refusing to comply with the culture of separation, scarcity and supremacy, and imagining something better. Collective well-being is big enough to hold all of us. It's not a trade-off between your personal well-being and our collective well-being. It's just more.*

---

* My favorite books that examine the intersection of wellness and social justice are *Skill in Action: Radicalizing Your Yoga Practice to Create a Just World* by Michelle C. Johnson and *Radical Dharma: Talking Race, Love, and Liberation* by Rev. angel Kyodo williams, Lama Rod Owens, and Dr. Jasmine Syedullah.

PERSONAL INQUIRY

Tension is my teacher. Whenever I come up against a place in my body that is tight, like my hamstrings or hips, I know it's an opportunity to work with resistance. I go gently as I feel my way into the tight places, old wounds hardened into tension and armor. Instead of pushing up against the resistance, I listen for what it is trying to tell me. I have learned to appreciate discomfort, to investigate it with curiosity, to trust that it has purpose on my journey. I ask, "What is behind the shields I carry? What am I trying to defend? What does this part of me need to soften and release?" The more I am able to be *with* my tension and not *against* it, the more it loosens its grip on me. Then I can receive the wisdom of uncomfortable—yet deeply necessary—inquiries.

- What were you taught about privilege and entitlement growing up?

- How have your race, class, gender, abilities, sexual orientation, and other identities impacted your well-being?

- In what ways are you advantaged and harmed by the dominant culture of wellness?

- Have you been silent or complicit in perpetuating the well-being gap? If so, how?

- What is your role and responsibility in closing the well-being gap?

- What does an everyday practice of equity and justice look like?

Democratizing Well-Being for All

Once I realized that my well-being was bound up with others', the yoga got real. I realized there was no solution to the problems we face that could be realized within the four corners of my mat. There was no meditating away poverty or racism. There was no manifesting peace and an end to suffering without getting explicitly engaged and political in the world. And that's when my practice became activism. No longer did my practice look like perfecting my pigeon pose. Rather, it looked like hitting the streets in solidarity with fast-food workers fighting for a living wage; it looked like confronting hunger and houselessness in my backyard of San Francisco; it looked like organizing and educating yogis on social justice issues; it looked like getting out the vote. Real wellness is wholeness—not only does it embrace the whole of who we are individually, but it demands the whole of who we are together. It is a collective practice that requires resistance and resilience to bring forth the beautiful, healthier world that we are all worthy of.

The pursuit and practice of true wellness demands that we confront the structural and systemic barriers that are in the way of well-being for all. While we may not have chosen our history, it is ours, it is everything in our past that is being made manifest now. It is the distribution of wealth that contributes to poverty, it is property ownership that shapes houselessness, it is the location of pollution that disproportionately makes people with marginalized identities sick. If we understand that our well-being is bound up with each other, we have no choice but to ask hard questions about who gets to be well and who doesn't, to challenge the commodification of wellness that reduces it to something that can be bought and sold, and to insist that well-being is a human right, not a privilege.

The politics of wellness are playing out all around us and are more proximal than you might think. They are reflected in how we price yoga classes, in who is in the front of the room, in how we pay and protect teachers and staff, in how we label bathrooms by gender, in whose bodies we choose to represent "wellness" in imagery and advertising. But wellness is also present in broader policies that ensure people have access to housing and healthcare, in workers' pay and protections, in economic policies that redistribute wealth, in antidiscrimination laws that protect people's dignity and expression, and in reparations for past harms. It's in how we vote and organize around the people and policies that reflect our values and our commitment to one another. Closing the well-being gap is going to take all of us leaning in, disrupting unhealthy systems and democratizing well-being for all.

To democratize is to make something available to all people. It demands that the "decision makers" at the top actually are dependent on the cooperation of the masses. We don't look to elected officials, CEOs, celebrity teachers, or anyone but ourselves and each other to change the world. We know our greatest power comes from our ability to reach, organize, unify, and act according to our collective values. If our collective value is well-being, then that becomes the central organizing principle of our practice. Our practice gives us the tools, a shared language, brave spaces, and internal resources to confront some of the most difficult issues of our time and to work to create the conditions of well-being for everyone. It is the practice off the mat that understands my well-being is bound up with the well-being of everyone.

Instead of trying to make unequal things equal, equity demands that we give people what they need to be well. And to do that, we have to acknowledge the complex social, economic, and political systems that are shaping health and human suffering in America. Traditional public health and well-being regimes that dictate individual responses to complex, interconnected ailments are not helping. They say eat clean, exercise more, block free radicals, buy organic, and avoid inflammation-causing foods, reinforcing the myth that we can become personally pure inside of the toxic soup. But you can't make healthy choices if you don't have healthy choices available. And if we continue to think about health and well-being from an individualized and isolated standpoint, we are going to fail on issues and we are going to fail each other. If we want to be truly well, we must seek to understand how the social world shapes people's health. Equity in wellness is the reorganizing and redistributing of power, resources, and access to overcome the cultural and structural barriers to well-being.*

But some even argue that equity is not enough because it is still working inside a structure and system that is broken (by design). Justice takes it a step further by challenging us to dismantle the systems that created the problem in the first place—systems of power that reinforce the oppression of marginalized groups while elevating dominant social groups. Justice is civil disobedience and nonviolent action that disrupts business as usual. It is organizing people and directing collective power toward advancing equitable programs and policies. It is centering the voices and leadership of those who are most marginalized, because they know best how to create a system that works for everyone. And it is voting in people who embody equitable values and voting out tyrants.† Because equity understands that we all need different things to thrive, it demands that our systems be relevant to all people and allow for radical self-determination. While equity makes space for everyone in this work, it also affirms that we have unique roles and responsibilities in advancing the conditions of well-being that work for everyone.

True well-being starts with the understanding that we are interdependent—that there is no separation between ourselves, one another, and the planet—and therefore our well-being is mutual and bound. That is not to say what it means to be well is the same for each of us. But it does demand that we fight for the conditions that enable people to thrive on their terms. Only together can we go toward the hard-to-look-at truth of our people and planet, the unknown and uncertain future that is in front of us. And when we reclaim well-being, when we say everyone deserves conditions that enable them to be well, then we can work together to ensure that no one is left behind and everyone can live up to their full potential.

---

* Reclamation Ventures is an impact investing fund dedicated to supporting the development and growth of historically excluded entrepreneurs in wellness: www.reclamationventures.co.

† To learn more about democratizing well-being and how to get engaged in creating the social and political conditions that enable everyone to thrive, check out www.ctznwell.org.

COLLECTIVE PRACTICE: LOCATE YOURSELF IN PROXIMITY TO POWER AND PRIVILEGE

Each of us has a social location that reflects our place or position in history and society related to categories of difference (race, gender, class, age, disabilities and abilities, sexual orientation, geographic location, social group memberships, etc.). These identities predispose us to unequal roles within the dynamic system of oppression. They are not a reflection of our worth but of the value assigned to these groups by society. Understanding our social location allows us to become more aware of our unique proximity to power and privilege so that we can more skillfully show up in relationship and collective action. Here's how it works:

1. Consider which identities within each social-group membership are more privileged and oppressed in society.

2. Then determine your location within each category of difference along the spectrum in proximity to privilege (center) or oppression (margins).

3. When you've completed the wheel, draw a line connecting each dot to give you a more holistic sense of your social location as it reflects the aggregate of your identities.

Note: There are many different sites of privilege and oppression that are not included in this wheel that may feel salient and significant in shaping you and informing your relationships and actions. Categories of difference such as education, language, religion, inherited wealth, and incarceration (among others) are significant indicators of one's location and lived experience and can be substituted or added to the exercise.

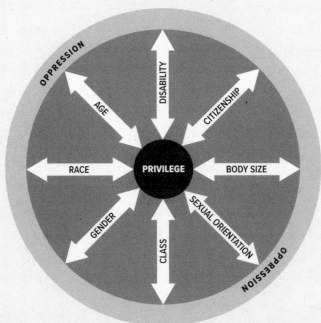

Social Location Wheel

Once you've completed the exercise, consider how your social location informs your role and responsibility in transforming our world into one where everyone can thrive. Consider the many circles and spheres of influence you move inside (professional, wellness, familial, etc.) and how you can show up and play your unique role in disrupting, divesting, repairing, or healing spaces. Locating ourselves gives us the awareness to show up in our communities with skill and impact.

CHAPTER 4

Perfectionists Anonymous

Perfectionism is the voice of the oppressor, the enemy of the people.

ANNE LAMOTT

I was born with something to prove. An unexpected blessing who arrived too early to a family that was not ready for me. While my parents' love for me was real, their marriage did not survive my coming. I felt the split down the middle, torn between two sides, two homes, two families, and two parts of me—the me that was innocent and didn't know any better and the me that had somehow caused their breakup. I felt responsible and committed to getting them back together, convinced that if only I had been a better student, more well-behaved, a good girl, we could be a whole family again. As it turns out, I would spend the rest of my life trying to become the person worthy of that wholeness.

Growing up in the white suburban shadow of Manhattan, I learned how to be a first-class overachiever—president of my class, captain of my lacrosse team, joiner of every club in the school, volunteer at local nonprofits, president of my Catholic youth club . . . you name it, I did it. Get good grades, be a great athlete, make things happen, serve others. It was how I was trained. And it made for a perfect onramp for a life in sales. Sales was the quintessential career for a relentless striver who needed constant validation and measurable worth.

And everything around me reinforced this. The voice of my family, my teachers, my community, my culture said, "If you're good, productive, and obedient, you will benefit." I was praised for my academic discipline. I was rewarded for my extracurricular activities. I was exalted for my ambition. I got friends and social capital. I got money. I got attention. I got love. Everything was for the sake of being seen and validated. Including wellness. Being well meant I had to have the perfect pigeon pose, the perfect Lululemon outfit, the perfect vegetarian diet, and the perfect social media image. If it wasn't perfect, it wasn't real.

But I was not alone in my addiction. Perfectionism was (and is) pervasive—reinforced by a demanding system that kept me in line and addicted to reaching, competing, defending, and hoarding. It was a relentless drive toward a never-ending destination that kept me deeply insecure and dissatisfied. From overworking to anorexia, I tried every which way to get a handle on it. But there was no winning at this game. Meritocracy and perfectionism were the price of entry into the "American Dream," a never-ending hustle toward an elusive destination.

And it just left me hungry, desperate, and wanting more.

Addicted to Perfectionism

Perfectionism isn't something we're born with; it's learned. Here's how it works: without knowing it, you practice, hone, and justify the skill until society pats you on the back for it. Before long, it isn't something you are doing but a way of being in the world—a chronic fear of failure that drives you to do more, better. So, you micromanage. You fix. You prove and people-please. You are always performing and assuming judgment. You set impossible goals for yourself and others. You criticize. You self-beat. You don't trust yourself, so you don't trust anyone. You live in fear of failure. You reject feedback. You can't tolerate mistakes. You refuse to ask for help from anyone. You worry. You get anxious. You beat yourself up. You get sick. You burn out. You lose friends. You lose jobs. You lose yourself.

According to Brené Brown, "Perfectionism is a self-destructive and addictive belief system that fuels this primary thought: If I look perfect, live perfectly, and do everything perfectly, I can avoid or minimize the painful feelings of shame, judgment, and blame."[1] It's not the same as striving. Perfectionism says that if you do not *do* it ___ enough (insert any adverb here: "smartly," "fast," "beautifully," etc.), you *are* not enough. Perfectionism is never about perfecting things or tasks; it's about perfecting the self. Which, of course, is not possible. And yet we can't help ourselves. Perfectionism calls to us like a drug. It tantalizes us with fantasies of satisfaction and achievement. It celebrates our futile attempts at attaining the impossible. It threatens us with shame and unworthiness. And it demands our obedience . . . or else.

But the perfectionist is, ultimately, doomed. Author Anne Lamott notes that "perfectionism is the voice of the oppressor, the enemy of the people."[2] It is an unreachable destination that keeps us stuck in the struggle with no hope of arriving. And it's expensive. It has cost me my body—forty-six years of pushing and perfecting has landed me with more chronic pain than I know what to do with. It has cost me work and professional development because of my rigid discipline, high standards, and unforgiving management style. It has cost relationships that have been lost to busyness, my sense of urgency, and relentless ambition. And it cost me my marriage because I could not believe in unconditional love and, therefore, I could not give it. Perfectionism has cost me much more than I've gained in its pursuit, and I'm only now learning how to recover.

The real function of perfectionism is to maintain control and power. It dictates what we get to avoid, what we get to feel, what we get to believe. It allows us to comply and uphold the limiting stories and lies that we tell ourselves about ourselves. And it operates like an addiction. Nikki Myers, yoga therapist and addictions recovery specialist, says that "addiction is the disease of the lost self" and that anything used to escape a perceived intolerable reality (like failure) is something that could possibly turn into an addiction.[3] Addiction is a constant and pervasive reminder that something is demanding our attention, and until we address it, we will remain stuck in suffering.* But the suffering becomes familiar, even preferable to its alternative. And we end up engaging in our own oppression and the oppression of others—giving in to a paradigm that says we are not enough and then profits from our not-enoughness.

Perfectionism thrives on not-enoughness—an impossible and unrealistic standard that doesn't just measure performance but measures our perceived worthiness. But feeling worthy is not just positive thinking, it's life or death. Melody Moore, licensed psychologist and founder of the Embody Love Movement Foundation, says, "At its root, perfectionism is about survival. It's a mechanism that we unconsciously solidify (often in early childhood) to stave off the terror of being too much or not enough. We believe, in our bodies and in our unconscious minds, that being 'perfect' is necessary for us to be in connection, to be fed, to be held."[4] That's why addressing perfectionism isn't as simple as changing one's mind. It must be dealt with in the body.

Body Wars

I spent thirty years of my life at war with my body. It wasn't enough to be healthy—I had to be skinny and fit, cute plus sexy, desirable but not slutty. I had to be what society told me I should be. And I was willing to do whatever it took to get there. What began as endless sports evolved into starving myself, working out obsessively, fasting, and eventually wellness. Yes, wellness—the socially acceptable (and celebrated) way to starve yourself and perfect your body. It was a perfect decoy for my eating disorder and my body dysmorphia. When I looked in the mirror, all I could see were the parts of me that didn't measure up to perfect—the love handles on my back, the cellulite in my thighs, the pouch in my belly, the sag under my arms. I didn't just hate my body, I punished myself for not being perfect— food deprivation (aka clean eating), violent workouts (aka hot yoga), forced

---

* Yoga of 12-Step Recovery is a holistic recovery program that "connects the dots" between the ancient wisdom of yoga, the practical tools of 12-step programs, and the latest research on trauma healing and neurobiology: www.y12sr.com.

isolation (aka silent retreats). And here's the kicker—my thin and able body was as close to society's standard as one gets . . . and I still hated myself. I asked my psychologist friend how you diagnose perfectionism that turns physically violent; she said it's called "dieting."

The roots of the word *diet* go back to ancient Greece and meant more than how one eats. *Diaiata* referred to an entire way of life that claimed that a healthy body and mind meant a healthy society (sound familiar?). "Healthy," of course, meant male, slim, muscular, and nondisabled. A few hundred years later, the idea (and ideal) took on new life in the "New World" when Protestant ideas of abstinence were gaining ground. What was once viewed as bounty and vitality in bigger bodies became sinful, indulgent, and gluttonous. This split was made even more apparent with the proliferation of print and the invention of scales. Thin would become one more toxic all-American ideal.

In *Fearing the Black Body: The Racial Origins of Fat Phobia,* Sabrina Strings says that the root of our obsession with thinness can also be traced to the transatlantic slave trade, which weaponized concepts of beauty and body type in the creation of a hierarchy of bodies. The racialized and gendered binary of fat versus thin "served as a mechanism for white men and women to denigrate the racially Othered body [and] also worked to police and applaud the 'correct' behavior of other white people, especially white women."[5] She argues that anti-fatness is not about "health" but about ways to legitimize race, gender, and class hierarchy. Da'Shaun L. Harrison adds in *Belly of the Beast: The Politics of Anti-Fatness as Anti-Blackness* that fatness and "health" are "used to tell Black fat people who and what they are, but they are also used to tell white people who they should not want to become."[6] The medical-industrial complex would institutionalize that ideology and justify the superior characteristics of the thin white body through pseudoscience and eugenics.* From there, an insidious culture of "weight watchers" emerged.

---

* For more on the correlation between anti-fatness and anti-Blackness, check out *Belly of the Beast: The Politics of Anti-Fatness as Anti-Blackness* by Da'Shaun L. Harrison and *Fearing the Black Body: The Racial Origins of Fatphobia* by Sabrina Strings.

Thin continues to be the standard for beauty, along with being white, young, cisgender, nondisabled, and flawless. And it sells. Marketers are notorious for selling aspirational and impossible images of the ideal woman. That's why over 90 percent of the models you see advertising clothing, cosmetics, and, of course, wellness products embody the thin beauty standard ideal. And it's working—more than 49 percent of adults claim to be preoccupied with weight.[7] In fact, fear of "fat" compels each American to try an average of 126 diets in their lifetime and spend more on dieting each year than on video games or movies.[8] But it's not just adults. Weight is the number one reason kids are bullied at school, and nearly half of three-to-six-year-olds say they are worried about being fat.[9] Let that sink in.

The "healthy eating" obsession is the latest in our pursuit of perfection. *Orthorexia* refers to an unhealthy fixation on eating "pure"—and it's on the rise. "Clean eating" has become code for food discipline and deprivation featuring macrobiotic foods, vegan burgers, bone broth, juice cleanses, and gluten-free snacks. Other self-care regimens encourage fasting and inhaling essential oils to suppress food cravings. In "The Thin White Men Who Rebranded Dieting as 'Wellness,'" in *Bitch* magazine, Virginia Sole-Smith describes clean eating as a phenomenon that "turns eating—an activity that, at its core, should provide comfort just as much as nutrition—into a contest of self-discipline and deprivation, of pulling yourself up by your Vitamix blender rather than your bootstraps."[10] But despite the lies that "health" and wellness sell you, your body size or weight does not determine whether you are healthy.*

Fat is not the problem. Thin privilege is the problem. Since the 1920s (with the rise of industrialization), mainstream US society has viewed thinness as a reflection of self-discipline, hard work, and moral superiority, while fatness has been equated with laziness, lack of self-control, and overindulgence. But as I discovered in my own struggle with body dysmorphia, you don't have to feel thin to have thin privilege. If other people perceive me as thin, I am thin. If I can walk into any clothes store and find items in my size,

---

* *Maintenance Phase* is an amazing and provocative podcast about wellness and weight loss, debunked and decoded by Aubrey Gordon (@yrfatfriend) and Michael Hobbes.

I have thin privilege. If I don't have to worry about getting a job or a raise because of my weight, I have thin privilege. Thin privilege simply means that your life hasn't been made more difficult because of your weight. It has nothing to do with the suffering or body image or eating disorders that thin people have experienced. It's just how society values thinness. Period.

But thin privilege doesn't work alone. It is the flipside of fatmisia, the oppression of bigger bodies. When thinness is uplifted, validated, and resourced, fatness is shamed, invalidated, and underserved. In fact, anti-fat bias and weight-based discrimination in the workplace occur just as frequently as racial discrimination. Fat bodies are portrayed as defective and wrong and yet capable of being cured if only the individual would try hard enough. It is a stigma that has a devastating effect. A recent study found that bias against fat people is actually a driver of so-called obesity. "When the culture and the medical world are constantly pushing the idea that 'obesity' needs to be eliminated, it's not the fat cells that are feeling that stigma—it's the fat people," says Lindo Bacon, author of *Health at Every Size*. [11]

But what if everything you thought about obesity is wrong?* Obesity, we are told, "is a personal failing that strains our healthcare system, shrinks our GDP and saps our military strength. It is also an excuse to bully fat people in one sentence and then inform them in the next that you are doing it for their own good," says Michael Hobbes, journalist and host of the podcast *You're Wrong About*. [12] Meanwhile, overwhelming evidence disputes the claim that an elevated body mass index (BMI) is linked to chronic diseases and a higher risk of death. America's obsession with obesity is not so much about health as it is about the culture of anti-fatness that diet, medical, and wellness industries profit from. Fat people are at risk of dying at higher rates than thin people, not because of their weight but because of a toxic system that fails to provide adequate care and denies people the conditions needed to thrive. Even as overt racism, sexism, and classism become unacceptable, anti-fat bias remains a valid stand-in: "a dog whistle

---

* *Body Respect: What Conventional Health Books Get Wrong, Leave Out, and Just Plain Fail to Understand about Weight* by Linda Bacon and Lucy Aphramor is essential reading to debunk myths and unlearn everything you were taught about health and fatness.

that allow[s] disdain and bigotry aimed at poor people and people of color to persist, uninterrupted," says Aubrey Gordon in *What We Don't Talk about When We Talk about Fat*.[13] We'd do better at improving health outcomes and life expectancy by addressing systemic issues such as racism, poverty, food insecurity, and access to healthcare.

You cannot wage war on fat without waging war on the people who live in fat bodies. "We can no longer pretend that being less likely to be hired or get promotions, being paid less, receiving biased medical treatment, being socially excluded and bullied are attempts to help people 'be healthier,'" says Bacon. "These are the direct consequences of living in a culture that vilifies and fears fat bodies and treats the people living in them as morally lesser beings."[14]

Meanwhile, anti-fatness is a great selling point for wellness. Movements masked in "detoxification" and "clean eating" just reinforce a culture of oppression that thrives on shaming and controlling bodies. It keeps us engaged in buying the image of "health" without understanding that healthy behaviors don't equate to aesthetic appearances. It empties our wallets and feeds a system that preys on our insecurities, and then it guts our emotional state by setting us up for failure over and over again. All in the name of perfection.

The Mythic Norm

I wasn't born wearing pink and loving dolls. I grew up a wild child, often found digging up the playground and storing pet worms in my pockets. I was curious and uninhibited, always up for an adventure and exploring the great big fantastical world outside. And according to my mother, I had a mind of my own. But when I started school, I quickly realized that wilding and worms weren't going to get me friends or favor. There were unwritten rules that said I had to look a certain way (wear pink dresses with bows in my hair) and act a certain way (play with dolls and be "girly"). And that's when I became obsessed with Barbie. Barbie represented who I needed to be to fit in—beautiful, blonde, skinny, fashionable, sexy, positive. And I wasn't alone. Ninety percent of American girls have one, making Barbie the queen of all dolls. Despite its iconic and aspirational status, Barbie didn't look like me. It doesn't look like most girls. It is a constructed and impossible image of a body that only occurs in approximately 1 out of 100,000 adult women (proportions so out of whack that she would not be able to menstruate or even hold up her head).[15] Barbie sales, on average, have grossed over $1 billion each year from 2012 to 2020.[16] But this is not about Barbie, this is about a toxic culture that sells us a mythical norm, manipulates us into wanting it, and then profits from our compliance.

Advertising and marketing (industries dominated by white men) shape how we see our bodies and the bodies of others. The avalanche of media we encounter on a daily basis, propping up aspirational images for all to covet, leaves most of us feeling insecure and inadequate. By most of us, I mean the 95 percent of us who don't embody the "ideal look" as defined by economies of exploitation and control. People of all backgrounds and genders internalize these perspectives, leading to physical, mental, and social consequences, such as body shame, social physique anxiety, reduced cognitive performance, eating disorders, and depression. Sonya Renee Taylor calls this the "Body Shame Profit Complex," the industry of beauty products that is valued at almost $600 billion.[17] It is a vicious cycle of control: keep us feeling bad about ourselves, then sell us a remedy that doesn't live up to its promise, which only makes us feel worse about ourselves . . . and so on and so forth.

We live in a world where people are constantly telling others what they can or can't do with their bodies. We're shamed from every direction—preached at to breastfeed, lose weight, act professional, dress appropriately. It is not just the private struggle with our inner critic, it is a public expression of how we judge each other and are perceived and policed by systems of power. From incarceration to disability violence to antiabortion laws to fat shaming, we are struggling to defend our fundamental right to bodily autonomy. Women are especially vulnerable to being objectified and governed by legislation, religious institutions, employers, family members, and culture. Messages of what bodies are supposed to look like and what we are supposed to do with them circulate in every aspect of our lives. We're surrounded. Society sets impossible standards and demands our conformity.*

---

* Some of my favorite feminist writers on radical self-love and body empowerment are Sonya Renee Taylor, Jessamyn Stanley, Lindy West, Lindo Bacon, Kimberly Dark, and Roxane Gay.

Even those of us who resist and reject society's expectations often secretly yearn to become the "perfect" woman. We make *Lean In* and *Girl Boss* best-selling books. We walk across hot coals with Tony Robbins for a breakthrough. We attempt to remedy our insufficiencies and defects through dramatic acts of self-improvement and self-deprecation. We work furiously to mold and contort ourselves into the ideal woman who has it all. We diet, we dye, we sweat, we push, we shave, we reach . . . only to be left feeling worse about ourselves. Rarely do we hear real stories about battling depression, caring for aging parents, borrowing money to keep up with the Joneses, faking self-care when we don't have any time, lying to ourselves and each other. But running ourselves ragged in an attempt to prove something or be taken seriously doesn't in fact work or advance women. We're set up to fail because the system is not designed for most of us.

In "Age, Race, Class and Sex: Women Redefining Difference," Audre Lorde defines the "mythic norm" as "white, male, young, heterosexual, Christian and financially secure."[18] Most of us lie outside of that mythic norm. And yet our failure to acknowledge the intersectional nature of our identities keeps us from uniting against the toxicity of white hetero patriarchy. Patriarchy is a social and political system of domination by which the wealthy, white, male ruling class has authority over everyone else. But often "everyone else" internalizes this belief system until it becomes the very strategy for maintaining our own subordination. In striving to overcome our oppression, we become the cocreators of the mythic norm, reaching for greater heights of achievement, until it betrays us. The #MeToo movement brought this home for me. It revealed that despite my ability to climb the corporate ladder and break glass ceilings, despite all those years of working hard and leaning in, despite my relentless ambition to be a career woman with a family, despite the belief that someday my children would have it better than me, I could still be cornered at a party, catcalled on the street, or raped.

The myth says that only when you perfectly perform the role of the perfect person will you be able to gain access to "respect, approval, education, jobs, equal pay, housing, physical safety, career success, love, space in our culture, bodily sovereignty, representation, justice if [you are] harmed, plus the full rights of citizenship," in the words of feminist educator Kelly Diels.[19]

All of these benefits are conditional upon your full embodiment and compliance with this externally imposed idea of perfection. The more impossible it is to perform this role, the more targeted you are for exclusion and oppression. Wellness follows this pattern, selling us on the promise of the perfect human and what we need to do (and buy) to fulfill that image. When we pursue perfection, we uphold a system that is designed to benefit some and discriminate, deny, exploit, and subjugate everyone else. We are implicated. But Audre Lorde reminds us that when it comes to the pursuit of these mythical norms, "each one of us within our hearts knows 'that is not me.'"[20]

Survival of the Fittest

I literally don't have a childhood memory when I wasn't performing for another's approval or striving and competing for external validation. What looked cute and competitive on the surface was often cutthroat at the core. I didn't just need to be better, I needed to be the "best"—to sell the most Girl Scout cookies, to run the fastest 40-meter dash, to get the part in the play. Whether I was conscious of it or not, every move I made was a strategic attempt to get ahead. It was a survival mechanism. I know that sounds ridiculous coming from a person with so much privilege, but the idea of rejection and failure felt like death—like a thing I could never recover from. It was perform or be annihilated. Playing the game became how I survived in a ruthless world made for human productivity. Which is exactly the point. Convincing even those of us with privilege that competing for approval is necessary for survival is an extremely effective tool of oppression. What better way to convince people with privilege that it will harm them if oppressed people get equity?

In a culture where performance, status, and image drive a person's usefulness and value, the quest for perfection isn't just desirable, it's essential. Perfectionism preys on our insecurities and sets us up in an impossible game of survival and achievement. But it's taking a toll. In a recent study, Thomas Curran and Andrew Hill noted an alarming rise of perfectionism over the last three decades.[21] Perfectionism, they claim, is how young people are attempting to feel safe and valid within a market-based society that puts enormous

105

pressure on people to demonstrate their value and outperform their peers. It is developed through the internalization of messages from their social environments, which informs how they view themselves, how they interpret self-worth, and how they relate to others. The result has very real and lived effects including anxiety, depression, suicidal ideation, anorexia, bulimia, agoraphobia, obsessive-compulsive disorder, insomnia, hoarding, chronic headaches, and more. The cause of this rise? Meritocracy.

In theory, meritocracy sounds fair. People advancing based on their merits, earning their place beyond their race, gender, ability, sexual orientation, and so forth. But we have never been on an equal playing field in this country. Not only does meritocracy reinforce the idea that one's success or well-being is an individual affair, but it makes people miserable and limits our imagination. While the impact of this kind of exclusion is hard to measure, increased inequality linked to meritocracy coincides with increased deaths of despair, the opioid epidemic, and the unprecedented fall in life expectancy among the poor and middle-class. The culture of productivity at all costs has many people working themselves to death for less money and benefits and a lower quality of life. Meritocracy isn't making us better or more perfect, it's just making us busy.*

And busy is my comfort zone. It is how I've come to understand my worth, my personal valuation in society. Like burnout, it is a badge of honor that I have worn with pride. It's status. It's working long hours. It's sending emails out at 2 a.m. It's returning work calls on a date. It's showing up late for commitments. It's letting relationships fall apart. It's neglecting personal health. It's forgetting Mom's birthday. It's making sure everyone else knows how busy I am. Because being busy is like saying "I'm important and valuable."

We live in a culture that rewards workaholism, relentless ambition, ceaseless comparison and competition, and producing at superhuman speeds. It is an unforgiving and elitist culture that judges anyone who is not hustling as lazy, stupid, and less valuable. Hustling is forcing, being desperate, searching for hacks, obsessing about the impossible. It is the gig economy that requires working endlessly to realize the dream while piecemealing together income

---

* To learn more about the false promise of meritocracy and how it feeds inequality, check out *The Meritocracy Trap* by Daniel Markovits.

from odd jobs and navigating bad, if any, health insurance. Hustling the dream looks good in theory. It sells us flexibility and freedom, which feels more like chronic anxiety and desperation. And corporate America is capitalizing on it. Fiverr, the freelance marketplace, targets the hustler's spirit in its advertising: "You eat a coffee for lunch. You follow through on your follow through. Sleep deprivation is your drug of choice. You might be a doer."[22]

And America loves a doer. No large country in the world averages more hours of work a year than the US. According to a Pew Research report, having a job they enjoy ranked higher than any other priority among young people, including helping others in need, getting married, and being kind.[23] And yet the more hours we work—the more efficient and productive we prove ourselves to be—the worse our jobs become. In the past four decades, most Americans have seen stagnant to decreased wage pay (despite an increase in productivity), eroding benefits (including healthcare, disability, paid family leave), and disappearing pensions (ranking the US near the bottom among industrialized countries that provide workers benefits).[24] At the root of this, says Jia Tolentino, "is the American obsession with self-reliance, which makes it more acceptable to applaud an individual for working himself to death than to argue that the individual working himself to death is evidence of a flawed economic system."[25] Meanwhile the highest earners are winning big, with wages up 138 percent since 1979.[26] Despite this, we stay in the hustle for fear of the alternative. We blame ourselves for not working hard enough. We work harder, for less. We identify with our work. We *are* our work.

Capitalism over Care

I was good at climbing the corporate ladder. Groomed from birth to compete and perform, I found my specialty in sales. There I would get lost in endless proving and quantifiable outputs. Sales was not just a job; it was a culture of manipulation and winning at all costs. One of the things that stuck to me from my sales training was the idea that you have to sell the client a need that they don't know they have. I was taught to expose their pain points and vulnerability and sell them the solution. And when I made the move from corporate sales to wellness "advocacy," it wasn't much different. But this time not only would I evangelize the benefits, I had to model the aspiration, which only reinforced my perfectionism and enabled my eating disorder. On the surface, wellness seems like it's filling a void left by an inadequate medical system. Look deeper, and the wellness industry reveals itself as just another business model based on grinding you down and building you back up again. There's a word for that: capitalism.

Capitalism is the religion that is at the core of all this—a chronic system structured around the institutions of private property, wage labor, and profits. It tells us that through competition the focus of supply and demand will find balance naturally and that the market is an objective and efficient place to determine and meet human needs. While capitalism has undergone many iterations over the centuries, from agrarian capitalism to industrial capitalism to free market capitalism, it consistently gives preference to production by any means necessary, placing competition above cooperation and profits over people. All of which is a part of a larger, dominant economy that is based in extraction. The purpose of an extractive economy is the "accumulation, concentration and enclosure of wealth and power" that goes all the way back to the wound of separation that resulted in genocide, the dispossession of Indigenous Peoples, chattel slavery, and the wholesale degradation of our natural environment.[27]

In this economy, we humans become our own extractable resource through the coercion and exploitation of our labor. We are only as good as the value we offer back to the market. And it fuels a conditional mindset that if we are more productive, we are more worthy; if we become more efficient, we can become more free. The myth of wellness builds on this ideology by trying to convince us that we are not human—that to be human, vulnerable, and needy is wrong. It tells us that we are objects to be perfected, to be optimized, to produce "health" for ourselves. But we have needs. We are not machines.

Whether you are making a killing or struggling to make a living, capitalism is making everyone sick. Consumerism gets us to buy into the idea that "the only way to be happy is to buy happy" and accumulate more things.[28] It indoctrinates us into an ideology of scarcity and an insidious sense of not-enoughness. Scarcity is manufactured and perpetuated by dominant economic systems through an inequitable distribution of resources to those at the top, lack of investment in meeting human needs, ruthless exploitation of nature, and waste of natural and human resources.* Capitalism is rigged for scarcity. And it doesn't just impact us physically, it impacts us emotionally. The contradiction of capitalism is that while it invites us to believe that abundance is our birthright (therefore enabling a history and culture of endless expansion and exploitation), it also states unequivocally that we cannot afford to care for the planet and all its people.

Scarcity drives the hierarchy of bodies that determines who gets cared for and who doesn't. Over the past few decades, a significant number of Americans have been trapped in low-wage jobs, with insecurity around food, housing, and healthcare, making it nearly impossible to get out of poverty. The federal minimum wage is still $7.25 an hour (since 2009), equivalent to $14,500 per year (well below the poverty line). In fact, today's average hourly wage has about as much purchasing power as it did in 1978.[29] Paid leave in the US is also among the worst in industrialized countries, often forcing workers to choose between their health and their work.[30] This was never more apparent than during the COVID-19 pandemic, when economic relief was conditional based on one's employment, not one's suffering or the severity of need. Worse, the price of being "essential" during a pandemic is that such workers (who are disproportionately people of color) are more likely to get sick and die due to financial insecurity, lack of paid leave, and lack of personal protective equipment (PPE).[31] Essential workers are called "heroes," but in most cases they're paid like shit, get no paid sick leave, and are denied basic human protections like PPE and healthcare— praised as essential but treated as disposable, all in the name of capitalism.

But they're not the only ones exploited by capitalism. In her book *How to Do Nothing: Resisting the Attention Economy*, author Jenny Odell notes that "much socially necessary work is ignored or devalued as caregiving, a gendered afterthought to the real dynamics of the economy when in reality no shared life could do without it."[32] Take stay-at-home parents, childcare workers, and elder caregivers—all invisible in a system that only cares

---

* For a more complex (and accessible) analysis of capitalism, I recommend *A People's Guide to Capitalism: An Introduction to Marxist Economics* by Hadas Thier.

about production. But no matter how much we produce, the cost of living continues to go up for working people while corporations rake in profits. The problem isn't productivity, it's that profits are being hoarded by an elite few. And the rest of us are left fighting for leftovers.

Fundamental to capitalism's ideology is the belief that there is not enough to go around, so life is a zero-sum game: in order for some to win, others have to lose. Scarcity is a part of our evolutionary history, when there was a very real gap between limited resources and abundant needs. But that no longer exists for a majority of people. We are now able to provide enough food, water, shelter, and medical care for everyone, if we chose to do so. The problem is not scarcity, it's distribution. Capitalism needs us to believe that there are too many people to care for and too little resources to share. It also demands that we, the workers, produce goods and services as quickly and efficiently as possible to be sold on the market. Failing to meet these conditions has very real consequences for workers. Throughout history the people deemed less productive have not only been disadvantaged in a for-profit system, they have been systematically eradicated through sterilization, institutionalization, and criminalization.

Which brings us back to ableism. Ableism is part and parcel with capitalism in how it enables production at all costs by rejecting workers who require accommodations. According to abolitionist organizer Talila "TL" Lewis, "This form of systemic oppression leads to people and society determining who is valuable and worthy based on a person's appearance and/or their ability to satisfactorily (re)produce, excel and 'behave.'"[33] And disabled people are often rejected from the workforce before they're even given a chance. "The capitalist needs the average worker to produce commodities—that is, goods and services to be sold on a market... If a worker is too slow and cannot meet these requirements, the capitalist loses time that could be adding more value for himself," says writer Chris Costello. "But there is a contradiction here: although capitalism rejects disabled workers, the system also disables workers."[34] That leaves 70 percent of disabled people out of work in the US, and many more struggling to survive.[35]

Capitalism does not care about people; it cares about productivity and profits, and anything that gets in the way of that is a problem to be dealt with, cured, or disposed of. But as writer and journalist Johann Hari notes: "You aren't a machine with broken parts. You are an animal whose needs are not being met."[36] Which begs the question: who would we be and what would be possible if we had what we needed to thrive, not because we are perfect or productive, but because we are human and worthy of well-being? And what would be possible if we centered care over capitalism?

RECOVERY

In a society that profits from your self doubt, liking your-self is a rebellious act.

CAROLINE CALDWELL

If I could go back and tell my teenage or twentysomething self one thing, it would be "*eat!*" I mean that literally of course—enjoy food, explore different tastes, fuck calories, don't skip the bread, trust your body, let it change, and eat anyway. But I also mean "eat" metaphorically. When I think back to all the things I deprived myself of—people I didn't meet, jobs I didn't apply for, experiences I denied myself, partners I wouldn't let myself love, life I didn't live—it was all because I didn't believe I was good enough or deserving of it. I was starving for connection and validation and was looking for it in all the wrong places. But despite my relentless driving, I would soon learn worthiness was not something to be earned but something to be believed.

Inevitably, perfectionism would betray me. Perfectionism is just shame masquerading as discipline. Inside the delusion of shame and not-enoughness was a world of hurt—chronic burnout, perpetual injuries, broken trust, failed relationships. Perfectionism wasn't making me better; it was making me miserable. I think back to all the time and energy that I invested in proving and performing when I could have been loving, connecting, and creating. The cost of my addiction was irreparable, but the choice to do something different, to own my imperfections and appreciate my worth without conditions, was profoundly shifting.

When I chose to say "Enough!"—enough to proving and playing the part, enough to denying myself nourishment and support, enough to desperately reaching for an impossible destination—I realized that I was not alone. We are all situated inside of this story that tells us we are not enough, that there is not enough to go around. Entire industries and systems are constructed to keep us afraid of lack and addicted to wanting more. It's a vicious cycle that keeps us dissatisfied—and keeps us stuck. But when we break with scarcity within ourselves, we discover a world of possibility for ourselves and one another.

Waking up to the lie of perfectionism is the first step toward liberation. We were born into a toxic world, raised in a culture that thrives off of our belief that we are not enough and profits off of our obedience to perfection and productivity. It is a system that takes more than it gives, keeping us in a perpetual state of striving and reaching for the impossible. There is no being perfect, there is only being human. But when we reject the lie—when we trust in our inherent worthiness and share ourselves out of generosity, not scarcity—then we can break free from capitalism's grip and live into our generative potential.

Healing invites us to declare our enoughness and reclaim the worthiness and dignity inherent to who we are. It means confronting the lies that we tell ourselves about who we are supposed to be and liberating ourselves from society's unrealistic standard of perfection. It challenges us to question where we are operating from scarcity, both within ourselves and within the systems we are a part of. When we remember that we are already whole, enough, significant, and worthy, we can imagine a world beyond proving and performing—a world where we are seen and valued simply because we are.

Detoxing Not-Enoughness and Scarcity Mindset

Hi, my name is Kerri and I'm a recovering perfectionist. This addiction keeps me striving toward unachievable and impossible goals. I hide inside my fear of failure. Busyness and workaholism serve as my socially acceptable cover. The belief that I am not good enough is a pull I have to negotiate and navigate every day. It is a choice, but it is also an indoctrination in a capitalist system that tells me I'm unworthy if I'm not perfect, productive, and always improving. Perfectionism is a lie; I know this. But when I forget—when I'm not paying attention—I will do just about anything to achieve the impossible. And thus goes the never-ending, no-winning, relentless cycle of scarcity.

Scarcity is such an enormous and all-consuming ideology that no matter how far I traveled on my journey, it always followed. From my suburban upbringing to corporate America to wellness advocacy, the hustle was there reminding me of my inadequacy and pushing me to do more. Being overworked, exhausted, and busy was a badge of pride. And feeling chronically unsatisfied was my state of mind. It was, and still is, the pervasive backdrop of a culture that thrives off our striving and keeps us distracted along the way. I was so busy proving myself, doubting myself, busying myself to death that I failed to see that there was no winning at this game, that it wasn't me that was toxic but the system of scarcity that could never get enough—a system that continued to take more and more while giving less and less. And I knew that I, we, deserved better.

Scarcity is just one more social construct (it's not real) that shapes our unconscious perceptions and drives our behaviors. Eventually we project our ideas of scarcity internally and begin to perceive ourselves as measurable and commodified. These views are deeply scripted within us, narrated by a system that benefits from our not-enoughness and relentless striving. When we don't feel valued, we don't feel satisfied. It keeps us trapped by producing an insatiable sense of needing more—more money, more material goods, more validation, more status, more everything. "Even when the game is going our way, we often feel a nagging disconnect," says Lynne Twist, author of *The Soul of Money*, "the gap between the way we imagine life should be and the way we are living it, under a daily pressure to earn more, buy more, save more, get more, have more and be more."[37] It situates us in this perpetual in-between state—we're "here" but we want to be "there." Here is lacking, it is not good enough, it is imperfect and unsatisfactory. There is not just aspirational; it is often idealistic and impossible. The cycle leaves us perpetually unsatisfied and hustling for more.

I was raised by a badass single mother who wanted me to have everything but refused to give it to herself. At twenty-four, she was raising a two-year-old, working nights, and going to school during the day. I watched her boldly hustle for the dream and sacrifice everything to give me the life she didn't have. My memories of her are a blur of her running from one place to the next, doing everything for everyone else, never complaining and never satisfied. She was a super woman. But in doing it all, she neglected the most important person of all: herself. While I inherited her work ethic and service to others, I also learned to neglect myself—to give and strive for some mythical future state when I would finally be worthy of receiving. It was "I'll buy the dress when I lose ten pounds" or "I'll go on vacation when I get that promotion" or "I'll believe in myself when I've reached 10K followers on Instagram." So much time wasted on not feeling good enough, so much energy spent on reaching for the impossible, and so much that I love lost in not acknowledging what was there all along.

When "not enough" becomes the default setting in our lives, it not only informs our lives but informs how we perceive and serve others' needs and well-being. The lack we feel within ourselves gets projected out onto everyone and everything else. Consider: How do you feel when peers get promoted? Do you compare your lifestyle to other people's? Are you constantly dissatisfied by what you have and what you don't? Are you waiting for the "right job" or the "right conditions" to do what is important to you? The delusion of scarcity is one in which someone is either higher or lower, more or less, perfect or inadequate, enough or not enough. It pits us against one another, forcing us to compete and protect our piece of the pie. But no one loses anything when someone lives into their wholeness. It's not a zero-sum game. We are simply human beings being human in a compromised world.

Perfectionism is a lie intended to keep us struggling in shame and scarcity—and moreover to keep us complicit in upholding systems of exploitation and extraction. Everything that we allow when we don't feel that we are enough not only harms us personally but also contributes to the cycle of oppression that is threatening our collective survival. Shame is political. It fuels the all-American obsession with being perfect, skinny, productive, and well; it is also the driving force behind a system that thrives on controlling bodies to keep people performing their roles in the dynamic systems of oppression. Healing is taking an honest look at the role we play in our own suffering and the suffering of others. Whether we like it or not, there is no escape from these systems, there is no perfect way of being, no clean lifestyle that allows us to transcend the toxicity of our culture. The world is a fucked-up mess, and no amount of purity and perfectionism is going to fix it.

In her book *Against Purity: Living Ethically in Compromised Times*, Alexis Shotwell argues that individual attempts at personal purity and perfectionism are not just impossible, they are also inadequate in responding to the overwhelming and complex issues we are facing.[38] Yet so often our immediate reflex in the face of that which we cannot control collectively is to try and control it personally by perfecting and purifying our individual lives; like if we just worked better or lived cleaner, we'd be able to arrive in a better place. To bring about less suffering and more thriving, we must accept complexity and imperfection as the natural basis of our lives. We are imperfect, imprinted by an unbearable past and unequal systems of power that are shaping our present reality. It does not matter how direct or indirect our engagement; we are embedded in it nonetheless. Once we become aware of this, we can take responsibility for our part in this mess and tell a new story of what's possible.

The aim of healing isn't to return to perfect. It is to return to human by embracing our vulnerability. "You either walk into your story and own your truth, or you live outside of your story, hustling for your worthiness," says Brené Brown.[39] Being at peace with our "selves" is remembering who we have always been, which unleashes our capacity to be our full selves and allows us to see and interact with others in their full capacity. All of us embody the complexities and contradictions that are endemic to being human. When we can cultivate a capacity to hold that for ourselves, we can hold that for one another. Only then can we experience our fundamental belonging to one another and to the whole of the planet.

To embrace this knowing—that we are all (though not equally) implicated at birth—is to engage from a place of acceptance and humility. We humans are already compromised. We've inherited and internalized systems of separation and supremacy that continue to run our world; every choice we make is imperfect and interconnected with everything else. And here's where it gets hard. Once you realize you're compromised and complicit, you have to deal with shame. Brené Brown defines shame as the "intensely painful feeling or experience of believing that we are flawed and therefore unworthy of love and belonging."[40] It's not that we did something bad, it's that we *are* bad. To admit you've spent your entire life working in partnership with a system that diminishes and dehumanizes people is heartbreaking, especially if you've continued to conspire with that system long after realizing it is not working for you. The only way to survive the shame is to stay busy, to make believe it's not happening, to justify it, to turn the other cheek. But shame never goes away no matter how hard we hustle to beat it. Getting free is getting real with ourselves.

That means recognizing that we've made mistakes, that we are a part of the problem, and that many of us still benefit. But it also means forgiving ourselves along the way. While perfectionism shames us into believing that we are fundamentally flawed and unable to reconcile, practicing acceptance and forgiveness teaches us that we can survive our mistakes and move forward. That's right. You don't need to be perfect in order to move forward. Abandoning perfectionism also frees us from the belief that we have to do everything ourselves. It liberates us from feeling like we need to prove ourselves to belong in the world. And it helps us remember our inherent worthiness, that which cannot be given or taken away. We are worthy simply because we are.

What was once an innocent need for me to be seen and validated as a child morphed into an obsessive pattern of perfectionism that evolved into workism and, eventually, into "wellism"—the unrealistic and unrelenting pursuit of trying to be well, pure, and perfect. All of which served as the ideal cover for my desire to belong and be loved. Perfectionism told me that I couldn't be loved, or love myself, until I was perfect, which meant I couldn't love anyone else either, unless they were perfect. Loving looked like holding people to impossible ideals until they loved themselves enough not to take it anymore. It cost me jobs. It cost me friends. And eventually it cost me my marriage. Learning to love meant loving myself despite everything.

In a culture that objectifies the body and commodifies the self, self-love is the biggest middle finger of all time—particularly for those of us who are taught that we are not worthy of love, or that we can only achieve worthiness through perfectionism or productivity. Self-love is standing up for yourself and your choices in the face of making people uncomfortable, disappointing others, and countering culture. It is rejecting society's standards of who we're supposed to be. It is refusing to give away our power for validation. It is recovering our body, mind, and soul from the toxic culture of perfectionism. It is self-determination for all bodies no matter what. And it is embodying a radical self-love that goes beyond other people's idea of perfect or normal or deserving. Radical self-love simply is.*

Striving for perfection and validation in a toxic world is who we've become. But love is who we have always been. Whole is how we were born. And being our authentic, messy, imperfect selves is enough. Self-love is how we call our power back and remember who we are and who we are to one another. It is reclaiming my wild and curious little girl self from the culture of Barbies and beauty standards. It is feeding my teenage body and soul the nourishment that it needed and deserved. It is letting myself off the hook for my parents' divorce and things that were beyond my control. It is giving myself permission to receive and rest (and wishing that for my mom). It is forgiving myself for hurting myself in my desire to be seen and loved. It is knowing that I cannot see another's worthiness and wholeness unless I see it in myself. And it feels hard and impossible sometimes, but it is worth it. I am worth it. We are worth it.

Our refusal to engage in the oppression of capitalist society is an act of resistance and radical self-love. We are more than objects of productivity. We are beings deserving of care. When we cultivate a sense of enoughness within us, we can more creatively and skillfully respond to the needs around us. While scarcity limits our imagination, dignity unleashes it, creating a capacity to dream beyond our limitations and toward cooperative models that take care of everyone.

---

* *The Body Is Not an Apology Workbook* by Sonya Renee Taylor is an awesome resource for how to work through internalized shame and divest from the system that benefits from it.

PERSONAL INQUIRY

In facing off with my inner critic—that part of me that says "you're not ____ enough" or "you're not worthy"—I have found that my greatest weapon is gratitude. For me, the practice is less about *doing a thing* (i.e., positive affirmations) and more about *being with*. When I sit with my judgmental self, I can bear witness to the longing that is underneath the mean thoughts. I ask "Is that true?" about the stories I tell myself about myself. And then I am able to discern the truth from the lies and see myself more clearly. That's when gratitude emerges. Gratitude reminds me that I am enough, that I have enough, that there is enough to go around. From that place, I remember that "I am already"—that nothing more is needed for my existence, that I deserve to be well and happy just because I am. From this place of knowing, I can dig deeper and do better.

- What is your relationship with not-enoughness?
- What did you learn growing up about your own worthiness and dignity?
- What has perfectionism or the culture of scarcity cost you?
- How has capitalism shaped your sense of self-worth?
- What boundaries can you have in work/life to protect your inherent dignity and ensure you are cared for?
- Do you know what radical self-love looks and feels like? If not, how can you explore that?

Recovering Dignity through a Culture of Care

The opposite of scarcity is not abundance; it's dignity. Therefore, to be against perfectionism is to be for dignity. Dignity in the way that my teacher, Miakoda, once taught me: "knowing that our best is good enough." It took me a long time to understand dignity in this way. I couldn't be available to it when I was committed to a practice of perfectionism. Even as I write about not being good enough, I'm questioning whether I am good enough. It comes up for me whenever I forget myself. It is only when I embrace my imperfect white privileged self that I am able to embody dignity for myself. Dignity, like worthiness, is inherent—it cannot be given or taken away. It does not play by the rules of supply and demand; rather it is measured in how people feel. When I am brave enough to own myself in all of my complexities, I am able to love myself.

Once we let go of scarcity, we can explore the world of dignity. Dignity cannot be quantified; it is not an amount of something that can be measured. Rather it is a way of being. The language of scarcity is: never enough, emptiness, fear, mistrust, envy, greed, hoarding, competition, fragmentation, separateness, judgment, striving, entitlement, control, busyness, survival.[41] The language of dignity, on the other hand, is: gratitude, fulfillment, love, trust, respect, faith, compassion, integration, wholeness, commitment, acceptance, partnership, responsibility, resilience. When you let go of trying to get more of what you don't really need, you are freed up to be generative with what you already have. Dignity flows from our personal sense of wholeness and serves our collective wholeness. It is how we define what is enough in the context of the whole. And it is how we build a future that takes care of everyone.*

In 1948 the United Nations declared that "recognition of the inherent dignity and of the equal and inalienable rights of all members of the human family is the foundation of freedom, justice and peace in the

---

* Another essential resource on dignity and mutual responsibility is *Dignity: Its Essential Role in Resolving Conflict* by Donna Hicks.

world."[42] But our capitalist meritocracy has reduced dignity to something people have to earn, while simultaneously setting people up to fail. Poverty pay and lack of workplace protections and benefits make it impossible for people to survive and move up in the world. Meanwhile, workplace policies protect profits, not people. Where is dignity in that? When we attach people's dignity to their job in a deeply unjust and unequal economic system, we betray them and their humanity. We objectify and reduce them to a product to be commoditized and exploited and then call it "essential." A system that exploits and extracts isn't broken; it was designed to do so.

In the absence of systems that take care of us, *we* must take care of us. Mutual aid is a practice and politics of collective care and responsibility. The concept emerged from a well-known anarchist socialist, Peter Kropotkin, in response to Charles Darwin's "survival of the fittest" theory that emphasizes competition over cooperation.[43] Mutual aid, on the other hand, is about building community capacity to meet each other's needs. And it's not just helpful or charitable, it's political. Mutual aid exposes how our systems not only are failing many of us but created the crisis in the first place. It encourages us to build horizontal structures of care and cooperation rather than relying on the state or wealthy partnerships. Mutual aid is a radical act of taking back our power and taking care of each other.

Mutual aid is not new, of course. Communities who have been marginalized by and excluded from systems of care have been figuring out how to survive for all of human history. Communities of color and immigrant, poor and working-class, and disability communities have long engaged in creative and subversive community care outside the system to ensure people had what they needed to survive. The Black Panthers built an extensive system of mutual aid including free breakfast, free ambulances, free medical clinics, free rides for the elderly, and free education for children. And the Young Lords, a collective of Puerto Ricans in New York, confronted oppression head-on and took survival into their own hands by commandeering an x-ray truck and hospital wing to provide direct healthcare to their community. But mutual aid doesn't just fill the gap. It also confronts the shame and stigma implied by capitalism—that our suffering is the result of our personal, moral failings as opposed to the exploitation and misappropriation of resources. And it calls us to confront our systems of scarcity, imagine and practice alternatives of care, and build a culture that doesn't leave anyone behind.

As the expression goes, we cannot solve problems with the same thinking that created them. It is essential for us to move beyond conventional thinking and ask critical questions about how different social systems can support or inhibit our human capacity for caring and creativity. In *The Real Wealth of Nations*, Riane Eisler argues for a "caring orientation" where the welfare and development of ourselves, one another, and the environment are highly valued.[44] In this world, we invest in human infrastructure and consider new ways of measuring capacity and growth. Conventional indicators of economic health, such as gross domestic product (GDP), give value to activities that extract and harm life while failing to acknowledge the work of caring for children, elders, and others in community and restoring the land. We need new, more inclusive measures that center the dignity and well-being of people and the planet.

Given the historical and present implications of the extractive economy, the consequences of which could destroy humanity, we must realign the economy with the healing powers of nature. That means divesting from the systems that have brought us to the brink of destruction and building a new world from the ground up. To do this, we must shift from a scarcity mindset to a caring mindset, from exploitation to cooperation, from hoarding wealth and power to collective well-being, from militarism to deep democracy, and from extraction to regeneration.* In this regenerative economy, work is not just jobs and material production—it is how we care for our families and communities, it is the contributions we make to our social and ecological well-being, and it is how we respond to harm

---

* Movement Generation provides a helpful analysis and strategy for how to go "From Banks and Tanks to Cooperation and Caring": https://movementgeneration.org/wp-contentuploads/2016/11/JT_booklet_Eng_printspreads.pdf.

and injustice. Essential to this shift is centering the sacredness of our relationship to each other and the world around us, where we are guided by our inherent dignity and understand ourselves as part of, not apart from, the living world.

To do this, we must create a politics of care where our systems and structures provide people with the capacity to care for family and contribute to our social and economic well-being free from domination and humiliation. It is more than job security and economic justice. It's making sure people have the space to have meaningful connection with their loved ones and with the world around them. And policies of dignity and care are already emerging.* Universal policies like universal basic income, parental leave, and subsidized child care would make working more sustainable for American families. Not only do policies of care move toward equal opportunity for workers, but they also provide essential support and connection that enable families to thrive. Like universal healthcare, universal worker benefits are designed to give people what they need, separate from what they earn. When we sever the link between employment and one's right to belong or one's right to thrive, then one's dignity becomes unconditional.

There is no perfect job, no perfect lifestyle, no perfect wellness regimen that will get us truly free. While these activities may seem "enlightened" on the surface, they continue to shore up inequality, erode social mobility, and create an ever more stratified society. Despite our relentless seeking, there is no relief or end of suffering that can be achieved when we disconnect from our pain and from one another. Recovering our dignity is inside-out. It is both reclaiming our self-worth as inherent and refusing to comply with oppressive systems that reduce us to inhuman objects. The more perfect world we are all yearning for isn't perfect at all. It's one where everyone knows that they are already whole, enough, significant, and worthy and we cocreate the conditions to thrive.

---

* For a deeper dive into the culture and policies of care, check out *The Care Manifesto: The Politics of Interdependence* by the Care Collective and *The Real Wealth of Nations* by Riane Eisler.

COLLECTIVE ACTION: CREATE A CULTURE OF COMMUNITY CARE

The many crises that have been escalating in recent years are exposing the inequities in our world, along with the very real need for ongoing job security and worker protections, universal health insurance, affordable housing, and more. But there *is* enough to go around; there is simply not an equal distribution of resources. In the absence of systems that take care of everyone, how can we show up to provide real-time relief to those who have the greatest need?

Community care is bringing people together to meet each other's needs. It rejects the lie that you're a failure if you need help. And it recognizes that our well-being is bound and, as humans, our survival is dependent on one another. Community care can look like a lot of different things: helping one another with childcare, mental health check-ins, financial assistance to those who need cash directly, food and meal sharing projects, disability allyship, legal aid and court solidarity, pet care and more.

Building our collective capacity to care for one another helps us reject the lies that we are not enough and there is not enough to go around. It reminds us that we are not powerless and we are most certainly not alone. Here's how to begin:

1. Take some time to learn the history of mutual aid practices and principles.* Mutual aid is more than reciprocal relationships of care; it's a political analysis and orientation. Get educated on things like solidarity

---

* Great resources on mutual aid include Dean Spade's book *Mutual Aid: Building Solidarity During This Crisis (And the Next)* and Big Door Brigade's Mutual Aid Toolbox: www.bigdoorbrigade.com/mutual-aid-toolbox/.

economies, affinity groups, horizontal leadership, anarchism, and Indigenous economic systems from which this type of work emerged.

2. Ask what needs and networks are already out there. Frontline communities, in particular, have extensive experience in responding to crises and caring for one another through collective mutual aid. It's likely that community-led networks already exist and that people are already engaging in some sort of support system where your unique skills and abilities will be useful. Mutualaidhub.org is an extensive aggregator of mutual aid groups around the country that you can plug into.

3. Consider what you have to offer. Redistributing resources (money/food) is needed in an unequal society, but there might also be other gifts (skills/knowledge) you have to offer that are needed for collective care. Mutual aid is an invitation to show up as our best selves and play our part in building structures that take care of everyone.

4. Be aware of how you show up. What is your social location and relationship to the people you are working with? Consider how you can skillfully show up to step up when needed and step back when you are learning. And follow the people who know.

CHAPTER 5

Getting Over Your "Self"

It is important for this country to make its people so obsessed with their own liberal individualism that they do not have time to think about a world larger than the self.

bell hooks

A few years after finding yoga, I had my "Eat Pray Love" moment. I quit the corporate world and decided to go out on my own. I was done playing by someone else's rules—checking the boxes and curating the all-American life. And once I let go of being perfect, I could start being me. Betrayed by the culture of productivity and perfectionism, I realized that the only way out was to turn inward and find my true self. So I set out on a new journey of discovery, stepping into my power and carving my own path. It was empowering but scary—I had no job, no security, no direction. But self-help was there to guide me.

My first self-help book was *A New Earth: Awakening to Your Life's Purpose*, by Eckhart Tolle. It came into my life to fill the void that ambitious striving had left, and I devoured it. What remains of the book on my shelf is a disintegrating stack of papers, broken in by tears and torn apart by sheer will. It told me to let the past be the past (good riddance!). It taught me the power of now and how to be present to my authentic purpose (ready for it!). And it said that I could transcend my struggle and become my most powerful self (finally!). Self-help had the answers I had been searching for. And before long, I needed a book for everything—what to eat, how to be grateful, when to sleep. Self-help had all the answers.

Anything was possible on the self-help drug. "The universe has my back," it assured me. "I can manifest a life beyond my wildest dreams," it promised. "Everything is figureoutable!" it guaranteed. I just needed to dare greatly, take an ice bath, and not give a fuck. Self-help was the essential handbook of my new life—an intoxicating mix of messages and life hacks designed to inspire change and strengthen self-esteem. It said, "You shouldn't be how you are—you should be better."

Except I wasn't feeling better, just more unsatisfied. My pursuit was relentless. Nothing and no one would get in the way of my self-improvement. I went to great lengths (and distances) to find myself until there was nothing left of my former life. All remnants of who I had been were replaced with high performance supplements and purpose-driven strategies. Eventually, my searching and seeking landed me on the top of a mountain in Peru after a seven-day trek. Exhausted, dirty, soaked, and sick with pneumonia wasn't the enlightened experience I had anticipated. What I thought would be a radical journey to finding my true self left me more confused, uncertain, and alone than ever. Self-help was an endless rabbit hole to an impossible destination. The further along I got on the path to self-actualization, the further away I felt from others. And I was about to learn that "happiness [is] only real when shared."[1]

Finding the Self

Finding the self has become an all-American fixation. We ask "Who am I?" and "Why am I here?" We claim purpose statements and start entrepreneurial projects, all for the realization and glorification of the self. We seek, we buy, we process, we manifest—anything to locate the most authentic "me" lurking inside of us. From finding ourselves to being authentic to living our purpose to profiting from our passions, the pursuit has become relentless. And it's not just inward. The demand to project and perform our best selves through social media has taken it to a whole new level. No longer are we finding ourselves for ourselves. Now we must perform the self for it to be real and valid.

The self-help trend dates back to 1859 when founding father Samuel Smiles wrote a book that became its namesake. *Self-Help* arrived during the change and liberation of the nineteenth century—abolition of slavery, industrialization, free-market capitalism, women's suffrage, freedom of the individual. People were ripe for Smiles's self-empowerment message of "heaven helps those who help themselves."[2] That message, rooted in self-reliance, would be adapted throughout the course of American history to tell individuals to "pull themselves up by their bootstraps" no matter what obstacles they faced (including systemic oppression). Whether it was in response to the Great Depression (Napoleon Hill's *Think and Grow Rich* and Dale Carnegie's *How to Win Friends and Influence People* remain on self-help best seller lists to this day) or in response to the gender pay gap (*Lean In*, ladies), the American answer to hardship of any kind has always been personal transformation.

But self-help went prime time in the wake of the Vietnam War, when people were becoming increasingly disillusioned with politics and losing trust in social and political institutions. It was then that we saw a shift from the mass sociopolitical engagement of the '60s and '70s to the self-fulfillment fantasies of the '80s. Alternative spiritualities like Scientology filled the gap, diet and exercise went mainstream, and South and East Asian practices like yoga and meditation took off. Even New Left activists began to defect to hippie communes and forsake the outside world for self-sufficiency. One such hub of alternative lifestyle was the Esalen Institute in Big Sur, California, a sanctuary that has been host to many of my transformational excursions. A breathtaking retreat perched on the cliffs of America's west coast, Esalen has its place among the origins of self-help and is considered home to the human potential movement (inspired by Abraham Maslow's psychology of self-actualization). From experiential workshops to psychedelic drugs to East-meets-West philosophies to commune building, the human potential movement met an increasing demand among people who were ready to unhook themselves from the hustle and discover their innate human potential.

This movement spawned the self-esteem phenomenon, evangelized by Esalen alum, human potential devotee, and California Assemblyman John Vasconcellos. "Vasco" believed that all that was needed to live well was to discover your authentic inner self, and he advocated for building self-esteem into the state education system. He claimed that low self-esteem was the culprit for an array of social issues including unemployment, crime, child abuse, teen pregnancy, drug abuse, and gang warfare (he even argued that it would one day balance the state budget). Vasco put self-esteem on the map, funding research, building it into legislation, and making it a pop culture trend that even Oprah endorsed.[3] America would become intoxicated by this trend for decades—it's been shaping the minds and bodies of millions of individuals and setting us up for the pervasive culture of self-help.

These days, the self-help movement promises to deliver you into greatness. From Tony Robbins's "law of attraction" to Rachel Hollis's *Girl, Wash Your Face* to Tim Ferris's *4-Hour Workweek*, there is no shortage of self-proclaimed prophetic voices selling you the keys to your own human potential. Memes spouting "Be bold," "Listen to your inner guru," "The universe has your back" are not only supporting the obsession with the self, they're validating it. There is even an anti-self-help self-help encouraging us to "not give a fuck" and just be our imperfect selves (of which this book might be one).[4] An $11 billion-plus marketplace in 2019 (projected to be $14 billion by 2025), self-help is built upon our addiction to self-improvement and our desire to mitigate stress.[5] That translates to a lot of books, online courses, and motivational speeches that have failed to dent a rising mental health crisis in the US that impacts one in five adults each year.

Nevertheless, realization of the singular and exceptional self continues to dominate, inspiring a marketplace of thought leaders, books, online courses, and self-help recipes that promise to deliver us from "mediocrity to greatness" (Lululemon's tagline).[6]

Selling Ourselves

The pressure to become an exceptional self is a very real and intense endeavor in today's self-obsessed culture. Over the last couple decades, the conception of work has evolved from "jobs" to "careers" to "callings."[7] We've come to believe that you can find meaning and transcendence at work. That you should persist until you find a job you love. That you should live your purpose. That you should be changing the world. We've become machines of self-optimization, sponsored by marketers, produced by social media. Although none of this is real unless we prove it out in the world.

Much of this performance, of course, takes place on social media—a platform from which millions of us sell our "best" selves and seek validation. Social media demonstrates our yearning for reassurance that we exist. We seek feedback on the images we are presenting to others, so that we can edit our way to a more attractive life. It serves to put forth a highlight reel of our best life—sans working eighty hours per week, navigating chronic exhaustion, dealing with panic attacks, wearing sweatpants, and living on popcorn. To be successful today, one is expected to perform one's newly reclaimed self-esteem into a measurable product for all to see. Social media becomes the vehicle through which all of our accomplishments are presented. The work isn't real until it's tweeted. The vacation isn't real until it's an Instagram post. The job promotion isn't real until it's on LinkedIn. The newborn baby or the engagement isn't real until we have proclaimed it on social media. Even our self-care has become a performance of achievement, not a reminder of our inherent self-worth.*

#Selfcare, a hashtag with over 50 million posts on Instagram, is the enormous marketplace capitalizing on our individual and collective distress.[8] It is the outsourcing of a culture that meets an ever-increasing demand to feel good and find meaning in a cruel and confusing world. Shayla Love calls it the "pull yourself up by your organic patent leather bootstraps" approach

---

* For more on the origins of self-care and the role Black feminist organizers have played in transforming how we understand health, check out *More Than Medicine: A History of the Feminist Health Movement* by Jennifer Nelson.

to health.[9] "[There's] the insistence that, in spite of all the evidence to the contrary, we can achieve a meaningful existence by maintaining a positive outlook, following our bliss, and doing a few hamstrings stretches while our planet burns," Laurie Penny writes.[10] It's a part of the fantasy that everything can be solved through the self, through individual measures, through the power of positive thinking. There is nothing inherently bad about self-care—it's essential to survival. But #selfcare is not that. It's just one more to-do list that we check off to demonstrate our productivity. It's companies selling cosmetics and juice cleanses and positivity journals that profit off of our perceived lack of well-being. And it's one more self-system designed to make us feel more inadequate and insecure.

Of course, my first default response to this trend is "that is not me." But in truth, I am the person who pretends not to care while obsessively checking for likes, comments, and shares. I use filters and angles because they look better. I say provocative things to get a rise (and followers). I "credential" people and things that will make me look relevant and important. I feel like a failure when my posts don't get lots of likes. I project judgment at others' feeds and fall apart when people criticize me. I edit and curate and put forth the very best version of me I can imagine. And worse, it is the version of me I want to be. But selfies aren't making me happier. They're making me paranoid. The truth is, social media does not care about our well-being. It only intensifies social comparison until we begin to prey on ourselves—comparing, contorting, curating, and cropping ourselves into perfect projections for all to see. And we have tech to thank for that.

The tech world has deep roots in the human potential movement. Between 1966 and 1973, America experienced the largest wave of commune building in its history. The "New Communalists" built communities that were a departure from the political collectivist spaces of the 1960s. They were retreating from politics and activism to build a self-sustaining hub of like-minded individuals that would shape a future of consciousness. Stewart Brand, founder of the Whole Earth Catalog, and others who came from the human potential movement evolved their mission to include personal computers as tools for the transformation of consciousness. Brand actually called computers "the new LSD" and imagined an entirely new infrastructure of

132

community connection. From there, Silicon Valley would be born.[11] Cut to the present, where we've experienced Russian bots, a Twitter president, selfies, and TikTok. While social media may not have created the ideology of "me," it certainly amplified it.

Today, the technology that connects us also controls us.* Platforms like Facebook, Twitter, and Instagram leverage the very same neural wiring triggered by slot machines and cocaine to keep us using their products and hooked on engagement.[12] The social approval we are so desperately seeking is being dosed to us every five seconds. AI-based algorithms predict what keeps our attention, manipulating us with behavioral science that hooks us into wanting more.† That's the point. We are an extractable resource, a data point, an impression, a product to be optimized and monetized inside a business model that is built on engagement and addiction. Americans spend about one-quarter of our time on screens, which has bled into our off-screen life in how we think about ourselves and our relationships. We start to conflate hearts and likes with real connection. And before we know it, social media has taken over our sense of self, worth, and identity. Social media is the drug and we are its users.

We're only now starting to understand the cost of our addiction to the almighty self. Teen mental health issues skyrocketed from 2011 to 2015, around the time that smartphones flooded the market.[13] And Facebook's own research confirmed that 60 percent of teen girls and 40 percent of teen boys experience negative social comparisons (leading to negative body image, increased anxiety and depression, and suicidal ideation).‡

---

* Check out the documentary *The Social Dilemma* and the podcast *Your Undivided Attention* featuring Tristan Harris for more on the dangerous human impact of social networking.

† In *Algorithms of Oppression: How Search Engines Reinforce Racism*, Safiya Umoja Noble challenges the idea that search engines (like Google) offer an equal playing field for people and ideas. For an overview of how algorithms impact privacy and equity, check out the Center for Democracy and Technology: www.cdt.org/ai-machine-learning/#content.

‡ Facebook whistleblower Frances Haugen's testimony spoke not only of the platform's harms to children but of the threat to democracy via misinformation and extremism. Check out her full statement: https://www.washingtonpost.com/context/facebook-whistleblower-frances-haugen -s-senate-testimony/8d324185-d725-4d99-9160-9ce9e13f58a3/.

There's also been a rise in narcissistic personality traits—such as vanity, entitlement, exploitation, authority, self-sufficiency, exhibitionism, and superiority—since the '80s, when the self-esteem movement hit its stride.[14] The ideology of the self-esteem craze would eventually be disproven when researchers concluded that it wasn't lack of self-esteem that led to aggression but high-self esteem coupled with a sense that one's self was threatened.[15] Our all-American fixation isn't making us better, it is making us bullies.

Cult of Individualism

Going it alone has always come easy to me. I think I learned it in the wake of my parents' divorce, that I would have to fend for myself by myself. So I pulled myself up, got good grades, escaped my small town, and made a life. When faced with setbacks, figure it out. When things get out of control, make shit happen. Self-help would entrench this mindset further. It said only *you* can change your life. Don't wait around for someone else to save you. You are the one you've been waiting for. In other words, suck it up and keep going. It was a recipe for a sort of self-reliance-on-steroids that would both make me and break me.

The emergence of the "modern self" accompanied the social, economic, and political changes that came along with the scientific revolution and an increasingly prevalent market economy that worshipped values of individual reason, self-determination, natural rights, freedom, and autonomy. Before that, many cultures valued the collective over the individual. But with the Enlightenment came a dualism that pitted man against the world, man above the world. This thinking, of course, inspired the United States to become "itself," a (stolen) liberated individual nation. "Give me liberty or give me death" became the war cry of our independence and imperialism and spawned a rebellious spirit that has morphed into American individualism and exceptionalism. Manifest Destiny took it even further, claiming that the US was predetermined and justified by God to expand its dominion across the entire continent, an ideology that would result in the displacement and genocide of countless Indigenous Peoples.

To understand American culture's fixation on the self is to understand how we have been shaped by history and culture to seek, nurture, develop, and manifest the self at all costs. It is the mythology of the American Dream that you can be anything you want to be. It is the "rags to riches" fairy tales that promise anyone can overcome impossible hardship. It is the rewards we are promised for pursuing perfection and achievement. It is the lesson of meritocracy: hard work always pays off. It is the psychology of self-esteem: if we believe in ourselves, anything is possible. It is the blame and shame that come with failure, and the belief that you could have done better. And it is the idea that personal freedom trumps everything else—including science, facts, safety, even human lives.

But this is not only about history. It's about all of us, all of us who have been indoctrinated to varying degrees in the all-American belief in self-reliance and independence. We value, above all other things, our individual freedom and the opportunity to live our best life—which many Americans define as paying low or no taxes and the right to carry a gun, or in the instance of the coronavirus, the right to not wear a mask. But it's not just MAGA hat–wearing, gun-waving so-called patriots defending their right to personal liberty despite the collective consequences. Wellness's self-help message is especially susceptible to conspiracy theories that exploit people's fears, promote pseudoscience and disinformation, and prop up unproven cures and miracle potions. Spiritual and wellness enthusiasts insist on their right to live outside the system, to pursue self-care over public health, to refuse vaccines, to escape to private homesteads, to opt out of politics, and construct alternatives to reality. All of which is leading us straight into extinction.

Individualism is the ideology that elevates the needs of the individual over the needs of the group as a whole. It emerged with the Enlightenment era just in time to shape a new American culture, where independence is highly valued, individual rights take precedence over the collective, self-reliance is celebrated, and success and exceptionality are worshipped. Individualism insists that people should be able to go it alone and pull themselves up by their bootstraps when they encounter setbacks. The "rugged" in rugged individualism refers to the aspiration and assumed ability to become totally self-reliant and exist without the support of communities and government. But the myth of the self-made man is a lie. No one got where they are without people and systems that supported them in visible and invisible ways too numerous to count.

This egoic ideology when crossed with capitalism bred a new Western worldview: neoliberalism. Neoliberalism is the agenda of deregulation, free-market capitalism, broad austerity, and the privatization of government functions. It is the culture of extreme meritocracy: everyone is in competition with everyone else, and your personal valuation is your worth. And it worships the market forces and strips us of the things that make us human. In a neoliberal world, we have become human P&Ls. Margaret Thatcher, who along with Ronald Reagan pushed for the neoliberal paradigm shift, said "Economics are the method. The object is to change the soul."[16] And that's exactly what they did.

Will Storr, author of *Selfie: How We Became So Self-Obsessed and What It's Doing to Us*, notes the significance of this shift. "The gamification of society triggered the 'Greed is Good' era, which represented a staggering transformation from the self of the anti-materialistic, communalistic hippies that had grown out of the mid-century's more collective economy."[17] The result was less support from institutions and the state, which put even more pressure on the individual. To survive and thrive in a neoliberal world meant you had to be better than your neighbor. It meant you had to be the best. It meant you had to win at all costs. And there's always a cost. The relentless focus on the individual, combined with a cutthroat economy, has elevated some at the expense of others. Our winner-takes-all attitude has increased the concentration of wealth and power in the hands of the 1 percent, leaving everyone else to find themselves among the leftovers. It is survival of the fittest, self-interest over everything.

Of course, the self is not "me" in a vacuum any more than the "self-made man" is solely self-made. It is very much situated, informed, and shaped by culture and systems. Storr adds, "When we're bathed from birth, in our particular economy, its values start to leak out in the things we say and do. Neoliberalism beams at us from many corners of our culture and we absorb it back into ourselves like radiation."[18] In other words, what we take in from our neoliberal culture is toxic. We give ourselves too much credit for success and too much blame for failure. And when we identify with our failures, we often descend into a range of dangerous mental health problems. The truth is, both our successes and failures are not ours alone but the product of so many factors that we don't control. And thinking we alone are solely responsible for who and what we are is ridiculous and completely untrue. The problem with individualism is that it ignores the fact that we're social animals. We live and survive and thrive in collective structures. There is no individual success story that is divorced from everything and everyone who touched one's story to make it possible. And it is our clinging to self-preservation and self-actualization that brings forth so much suffering.

Pat MacDonald, author of the paper "Narcissism in the Modern World," says, "Much of our distress comes from this state of disconnection. We have a narcissistic society where self-promotion and individuality seem to be essential, yet in our hearts that's not what we want. We want to be a part of a community, we want to be supported when we're struggling, we want a sense of belonging. Being extraordinary is not a necessary component of being loved."[19] And we are far from extraordinary; that's part of the disillusionment and anxiety. We humans are inherently imperfect works-in-progress who are wired for social connection. And yet we are steeped in a culture that is selling us the myth that the individual, perfect, exceptional self is the key to happiness. It's not.

Social Isolation

By my midthirties, I was living the dream. Girl leaves her high-powered job. Girl goes on a journey of self-discovery. Girl finds a spiritual path. Girl reinvents herself. By all measures, I was a self-help success story. I had launched a business, I spoke on panels, I was featured in magazines and on billboards, I was admired by others. So why was I so depressed? It was like the more I "found" myself in mantras and master classes, the more lost and alone I felt.

A paradox of our hyperconnected digital culture is that we increasingly feel more alone. Social media both brings us together and drives us apart.

Our need to differentiate the exceptional self is actually making us more lonely. We become pitted against each other in competition, trapped in eighty-hour work weeks, laser-focused on our quest for self-achievement and actualization. We feel dislocated from a sense of belonging and meaningful experience of community. Instead of trying to reconcile the alienation that comes with selfhood, dominant culture encourages us to take control and embrace our individuation. But this kind of social isolation is deadly.

Enter the loneliness epidemic. Over the last five decades, rates of loneliness have doubled in the United States.[20] Even before the COVID-19 pandemic, a 2018 survey of over 20,000 American adults found that almost half of respondents reported feeling alone, left out, and isolated.[21] We are losing a sense of connection and belonging that is fundamental to human thriving. And this loss has serious costs. Scientists have known for some time that loneliness is emotionally painful and can contribute to conditions such as depression, anxiety, and schizophrenia.[22] More recently, however, they have learned how destructive loneliness is to the body. In 2015 researchers at UCLA discovered that social isolation causes cellular changes that result in chronic inflammation, increasing the likelihood of serious physical conditions such as heart disease, stroke, metastatic cancer, and Alzheimer's disease.[23] Loneliness is considered more lethal than smoking fifteen cigarettes a day and raises the risk of early death by 26 percent.[24]

One of the biggest indictments of this toxic system is the opioid and heroin epidemic. Every day 136 people die in this country from an overdose.[25] Since 2002, the number of deaths by heroin per year has increased by over 500 percent.[26] What's driving this addiction? Isolation. While we cannot see social pain in the same way we see physical pain, its existence is evidenced in neuroscience. Both kinds of pain are processed by the same neural circuits. Opioids relieve both physical and social pain (the distress of isolation), making an obvious link between social isolation and drug addiction even more explainable. When we don't have the ability to authentically connect, to have experiences of belonging and transcendence beyond the self, we become vulnerable to seeking relief in all the wrong places. And it's no wonder, given the rise in digital consumption, hyperproductive lifestyles, a culture of self-reliance, and inequality.

As neuroscientist Rachel Wurzman points out in her TED Talk "How Isolation Fuels Opioid Addiction," the places hit hardest by the economy, where people are more likely to feel desolate about their situation, are also communities most ravaged by the opioid epidemic. "Social isolation acts through the brain's reward system to make this state of affairs literally painful. So perhaps it's this pain, this loneliness, this despondence that's driving so many of us to connect with whatever we can. Like food. Like handheld electronics. And for too many people, to drugs like heroin and fentanyl."[27] This was exacerbated during the quarantine of 2020, when we were forced to physically distance to slow the spread of the coronavirus. Disconnected from our lives and one another, many turned to Netflix and online yoga classes and TikTok for comfort and normalcy. But while tech and consumerism filled the void, "deaths of despair" soared.

While science continues to affirm that our well-being is interconnected, culture reinforces the lie that we will flourish in competitive self-interest and extreme individualism. But social connection is to well-being like water is to hydration. It just is. The idea that we are better off self-actualized and alone is absurd and dangerous. And while it's easy to point the finger at technology, its roots are more complicated—partly attributed to neoliberal economics that sells us on the idea that we will prosper through self-interest above all things, partly due to the ideology of extreme individualism, and partly due to the breakdown of social and civic structures. What's required is beyond policy change: a reorientation of our worldview—one that affirms our interdependence and the role of community in our personal and collective thriving.

Harvard scientist Robert Putnam wrote about the "end of community" in *Bowling Alone*, an influential book from 2000 that talks about how Americans have become increasingly disconnected from family, friends, neighbors, and our democratic structures.[28] Institutions like churches, unions, civic organizations, and schools have historically worked to challenge the myth of self-reliance; they value the well-being of the community over the well-being of the individual. But the role and power of these social structures don't have the same relevance they once did. Fewer Americans are religiously affiliated. Increased partisanship has driven people apart. The loss of union power has made it harder for organized labor to build collective power and social capital. Digital media is privatizing our leisure time. All of this works to reduce collective power, increase isolation, and prevent diversity of community and experience.

We've been stuck in a culture of social distancing long before COVID-19. The erosion of accessible community structures over the last few decades has left us striving for self-preservation above collective care. Individuals and communities have become more isolated and fragmented, breaking away from the social bonds of many aspects of life—familial, neighborly, religious, social, and civic. In the absence of community structures that anchor people in mutual interest and cooperation, a culture becomes vulnerable to the traps of self-reliance, self-interest, and even self-care. Reclaiming our individual and collective selves can't be found in self-help books and personal seeking; it can only be achieved through relationship and community.

The irony of American life is that our obsession with self and individual liberty has made us less supported and more vulnerable. All of the political freedoms we are supposedly entitled to as American citizens are useless in the face of the many interdependent crises we are facing—whether it be economic collapse, a deadly pandemic, or environmental devastation.

The only way to get free is through each other.

RECOVERY

It is in community and relationship with others that we locate a self that we can never find being isolated. It is in community and in relationship with each other that we come to know the consciousness and the spirit of God that is in each of us.

RUBY SALES

Right around the time of my self-help revolution, my marriage fell apart. No longer were we the people we had married. We were growing apart, and I was desperately trying to self-help save us. Much to my then-husband's dismay, I made him eat tofu, read *The 5 Love Languages*, do partner yoga, and chant mantras. I insisted I knew what was best for us and had the Truth-with-a-capital-T on my side. I flaunted my new practices, preached my enlightened ideas, and upended our life until it was unrecognizable. Not only was I determined at all costs to become my best self, I tried to drag him along for the ride. But I wasn't trying to help us. I was trying to change him. And after eighteen years of "'til death do us part," I walked away. I will likely never fully understand what went wrong or what could have been. I only know the pain that was left over in its wake. Divorce is like a flesh wound: a part torn away never to be retrieved. There was no praying away my pain, no manifesting love and light in the midst of so much loss. Despite my relentless attempt to find myself, I ended up more lost and alone than ever.

Looking back, I can see now my part in the death of our marriage. While I can't control how two people change over time, I can own that my obsession with finding myself and fixing us is part of what drove us apart. Self-help didn't save my marriage; it gave me an out, a way to bypass the beautiful and brutal work of being in relationship. So many of us attempt to engage in self-growth and -actualization in a vacuum. But we do not live in a vacuum. We impact each other and we are impacted by each other. True, integrated self-growth includes both self-acceptance *and* acceptance of others. I learned that lesson too late.

The idea that I am alone, that I can depend on no one, that I must fend for myself and by myself, has caused me more suffering than I can measure. It is the wound of my parents' divorce that drove me to become an independent, self-sufficient child, and it is the wound of my own failed marriage. But it is also the ideology of self-help that convinced me that I had the power alone to solve all my problems. I exhausted myself with morning rituals, checklists, confidence poses, journaling practice. Everything had to be optimized. Self-help spawned an obsessive never-ending battle to improve myself (aka perfection) that is never won. This inevitably leads to failure and pushes us further apart from one another. When we are stuck in our silos of self-improvement, we become cut off from the very source of well-being: each other.

Individualism sells us the lie that we are better off by ourselves. It convinces us that self-improvement is the cure to all that ails us. It says that needing help is a weakness and we should trust ourselves above all else. And it says that we are separate and exceptional beings that should pursue self-betterment at all costs. What it doesn't say is that none of your greatness would exist without the system of labor and exploitation that makes it possible, that your self-actualization is too often accomplished on the backs of others. And it most certainly won't admit that while you're finding yourself, others are struggling to survive much less be enlightened. Self-help is a part of the all-American mythology of the self-made man. But that dream wouldn't have been possible without the theft of lands and the exploitation of labor. No one gets anywhere on their own. Our individual and collective flourishing is only made possible by the many interlocking contributions that make society work.

What we are so relentlessly seeking is a purpose not for the sake of purpose, but purpose in relationship to the world. The human condition is one of connection and belonging. All of the crises we have faced—whether 9/11 or climate change or the coronavirus—underline the interconnectedness that has always been and the inadequacies of our self-oriented lives. We are not separate from the suffering of our people and our planet. Only when we can unhook ourselves from the demands of the self can we accept ourselves and embrace the true self—the self that is part of something bigger than the self. To do this, we must reject the lie of separation and reclaim our connection to ourselves and one another. In many ways, this detox is an invitation to come home to the truth of who you are as an authentic interbeing.

Finding Ourselves through Each Other

I spent most of my life in the delusion that all of my success and accomplishments were mine alone. That I had no one to thank but myself for who I was and what I had achieved. Privilege is powerful in how it reinforces our perceived independence and shields us from seeing the truth. It was only when I found myself in suffering that I understood who and where I came from. Whether it was in the wake of 9/11 or in recovery after my back injury or in the aftermath of my divorce, I would learn the hard way that I was nothing without relationship. And if it weren't for community and support, I would be alone and out on my ass.

Despite the costs of individualism, America continues to prop the self up above all other things. So many of us become accustomed to going it alone, doing what we want when we want it, defending and preserving our individual wants at all costs. We see it in the erosion of the social safety net, in austerity policies, and in the privatization of human resources that puts profits over people. We see it in a culture that convinces us to let capitalism run its course and that wealth trickles down to benefit everyone. We see it in the cries for freedom that project one person's right to own a gun over another person's right to live. And we see it in the "wellness of me" that keeps us gazing at our navels, believing that we are in control, and shames us when we inevitably fail to achieve the impossible. But it is this delusion that keeps us striving in isolation, being stuck and unwell.

Psychologists have long pointed to self-actualization as the pinnacle of Abraham Maslow's hierarchy of human needs. However, Maslow discovered later in his life that he was wrong.[29] There was, in fact, a deeper

143

motivation, which he called transcendence—a commitment to the greater good. "The fully developed (and very fortunate) human being, working under the best conditions tends to be motivated by values which transcend his self."[30] This theory went beyond the ego self to encompass our relationship to one another and the bigger world that we are a part of. Of course that is not the version we hear most often in the field of psychology. Nor do we hear that much of Maslow's work was influenced by the wisdom of the Siksika Nation (a part of the Blackfoot confederacy in Canada), who understood one's needs not as hierarchical but as circular and contextual at the levels of self, community, and culture equally.[31]

While seeking the self may seem innocent and well intentioned, its shadow runs deep in all of us who cannot see the "Self" beyond the self, who get stuck trying to navel-gaze our way to growth. This "small self" inspires us to turn inward as if we can articulate and perfect ourselves apart from the soup we are swimming in, but there is no enlightened state or transcended plane that is immune to the systems and structures we are steeped in. Rather we are a capital-S whole Self in deep interconnectedness with everything and everyone around us. There is no achievement, no superior state that can be accomplished without the support of invisible others. Consider who paves the roads to the yoga studio and the Whole Foods, who maintains the Wi-Fi signals that make it possible to post selfies and stream meditations, who farms and ships and stocks and sells the superfood that contributes to a clean and healthy diet. But it's not just the interconnected systems we are a part of. It is the people who raised you, the teachers who inspired you, the friends who have shown up for you when you couldn't show up for yourself. It is everyone and anyone who has crossed your path and shaped your life. The idea of the separate and exceptional self is a lie, because the experience of being a human living in community with other humans means that we impact each other and are impacted by each other. There is no getting around this; no clean-living solution, no retreat to which you can escape, no self-help hack can save you from the truth of our interdependence.

When we make the self the outer limit of our experience, we become ignorant to the way in which many of our identities are constructed for us, not by us. Our self-righteousness is unable to see beyond its "self" and, therefore, reinforces the illusion of separation and bypasses the reality of our differences and the wisdom of our interconnectedness. We are left with a deep sense of loss and fear that haunts the ego self. The real existential crisis in America is not who we are as individual selves, it's who we are beyond the conditions that convince us that we are separate and exceptional. That is the irony of individualism—our fixation with the "small self" (the self as an object that does not extend beyond the edges of our body) actually limits our human potential. It keeps us alone and isolated. It makes us reject our own needs and the needs of others. It sets us up for shame and makes us believe we are unworthy of belonging. And it denies our humanity. This small self isn't potential, it's prison. It is the worst kind of punishment. It's the life orphaned from its fundamental right to belong.

Healing from individualism invites us to examine our need to "go it alone" and see all the ways in which we are at war with ourselves. Our relentless yearning for the better self is often driven by a rejection of the vulnerable human self. We end up forsaking the parts of us that are flawed, imperfect, and not "normal." We don't trust ourselves so we don't trust others, tearing us further apart. This split not only works against our healing but inevitably sets us up for suffering and isolation. In *A Hidden Wholeness*, Parker Palmer notes: "We arrive in this world undivided, integral, whole. But sooner or later we erect a wall between our inner and outer lives, trying to protect what is within us or to deceive the people around us. Only when the pain of our dividedness becomes more than we can bear do most of us embark on an inner journey toward 'living divided no more.'"[32]

When I couldn't tolerate myself—the self that felt isolated and inadequate—I tried to construct something else, something other, some better version of myself. But othering ourselves or anyone else doesn't move us toward wholeness and liberation. It keeps us stuck and small in its attachment to form and actualization. It is an insatiable cycle of always wanting, never satisfied, and therefore chronically suffering. In my relentless seeking, I had forgotten the fundamental truth of who we are—that we belong to each other. Of course, we cannot see another's divinity (their inherent dignity and worthiness) without seeing that in ourselves; and conversely, we see our own more clearly in relationship with others.

Living from the small self doesn't just divide us personally, it divides us collectively. This form of othering is not as simple as liking or disliking someone; rather, it is the process of not seeing, really seeing, people in their full humanity and sacredness. Instead we often see them as competition, see them as different, see them as less than, see them as a threat. And from this place of othering come all forms of harm—harmful relationships across lines of difference, harmful laws that police and exploit bodies, harmful narratives that say who is worthy of belonging and who isn't.* Furthermore, this lack of connection isn't only harming others, it is harming us, causing psychological and spiritual suffering with very real consequences on our minds and bodies. To heal this, we need to reclaim what Thich Nhat Hanh calls "interbeing," or a sense of deep and authentic relationship with one another and the world around us.[33]

In the same way we long to be seen by others, self-awareness is the ability to see ourselves more clearly. It means asking questions that challenge and complicate our own truth. Brené Brown calls this "rumbling with vulnerability"—"having some critical awareness around the stories we make up, doing fact-finding, and getting curious around what we are feeling."[34] It's how we check ourselves and interrogate the stories that we tell ourselves about ourselves. This "interrogation" isn't about judgment or shame—those are just more weapons of division. Rather it is a willingness to be clear-seeing about ourselves, about how we have been socialized and shaped by a toxic culture, about how we have become separated from the truth of our belonging. But to do this sustainably, we must marry clarity with compassion.

Jack Kornfield said, "If your compassion does not include yourself, it is incomplete."[35] While the self-esteem movement breeds social comparison and narcissism, self-compassion generates inner worth and strength. Self-esteem is boisterous and fleeting. It deserts us when we need it most, usually after we fail to live up to our expectations or don't measure up to the

---

* The Othering and Belonging Institute is committed to expanding the circle of human concern. Check out their article "The Problem of Othering: Towards Inclusiveness and Belonging" by john a. powell and Stephen Menendian: https://otheringandbelonging.org/the-problem-of-othering/.

competition. Compassion invites us to expand beyond the limitations of the small self.* But it also entails a recognition of our common humanity—and the knowing that all people are imperfect, and all people have imperfect lives. Despite what we see on social media, most people are making a mess and fumbling through life. We cannot heal our way out of being human. Recognizing our shared humanity opens the door to showing up and growing up.

Understanding the compassionate self as part of the whole is what inspired self-care in the first place. According to Black feminist icon Audre Lorde, who wrote the words after she was diagnosed with cancer, self-care was protest, a way to protect Black women when no one else would. "Caring for myself is not self-indulgence, it is self-preservation, and that is an act of political warfare."[36] When we reclaim self-care in this way, it is a radical act of defiance in a system that only attaches worth to our output and productivity. Self-care, when divested from productivity and individualism, is rejecting the status quo and "overthrowing the systems that are designed to define, restrict, and police who you are."[37] It allows us to be fully expressed. It is resting.† It is demanding nothing less than what we deserve. Self-care in this way understands that there is no self that is separate, no care that is not collective, and no love that is conditional.

We are wired for connection. Connection is our true nature. Similarly, sociologists assert that the fundamental unit of human existence is the small group and not the individual. We are who we are because of each other. The lie of individualism is not just that we are separate exceptional selves, but that we can heal ourselves by ourselves. What I have come to learn is that no amount of self-inquiry, self-esteem building, or self-development would change me as much as I would be changed in relationship. My third-grade teacher who believed in me changed me. Knowing Joe and losing Joe on 9/11 changed me. All of the friends who loved me at my worst changed

---

* Kristin Neff has done extensive research on self-compassion. Check out her Tedx Talk on the difference between self-compassion and self-esteem: www.youtube.com/watch?v=IvtZBUSplr4.

† Rest is revolutionary in a capitalist culture of productivity and exploitation. Check out Tricia Hersey's Nap Ministry, Tracee Stanley's *Radiant Rest*, and Octavia Raheem's *Pause, Rest, Be* for more on radical rest and recovery.

me. Getting married changed me. Getting divorced changed me as well. I am who I am because of relationship. The self that I know myself to be has been shaped and imprinted by the people who have crossed my path. The "me" I have been seeking is really a "we."

PERSONAL INQUIRY

When I am feeling lonely and lost, I have learned to let the world in. Breath is the bridge that brings me back into relationship with everything and everyone around me. I begin by getting grounded in myself, letting wherever I'm at be the starting point. I follow the wave of my breath as it enters and leaves me. Breathing out, I let go of whatever is in the way of my truth. Breathing in, I let in the outside world. With each breath I expand my capacity to center in myself and expand out in relationship. I invite my senses to include more, noticing the sights, scents, touch, and taste of the dynamic world I am a part of. Eventually I experience myself not in the world but of the world itself. And from here, I can access my bigger "Self" in deep inquiry and contemplation.

- What cultural messages have you received about "going it alone"?

- How have you been shaped by the culture of self-improvement, self-help, and self-made?

- What has the myth of individualism cost you in your life?

- What have you learned about yourself in relationship that would not have been possible in isolation?

- What are some specific ways you can move from isolation to connection?

- How can you embrace your unique purpose, not in a vacuum but as an essential part of a larger ecosystem?

It was from this place, revealed to me through relationship and community, that I discovered my unique assignment in the world. My purpose wasn't about me; it was so much bigger. It is being a commitment to our collective potential, through organizing people and taking action toward a world where everyone is free to be their most authentic selves. It is confronting everything that is in the way of our ability to be our full and whole selves. And it is showing up in solidarity for the well-being of everyone.

Restoring Relationship through Solidarity

We are experiencing a crisis of connection on every level—whether we've become disconnected from our bodies, from one another, from critical social issues, or from democracy. And the social cost of this disconnection is playing out across the country, as evidenced in political gridlock, underfunded schools, economic inequality, gun violence, children living in poverty, deaths of despair, climate change, and more. Disconnection keeps us from pursuing collective liberation. It keeps the lie of separation alive. We may strive to become our best selves, but ironically we don't do that all by our "self." There is no self that is separate from everything and everyone around us. There is no pursuit of happiness or enlightenment that is divorced from our intrinsic relationship with one another. Reclaiming our relationality is how we recover from the wound of individualism and find our place in the world.

While individual transformation is the more popular conversation in the wellness world, we have already seen that the transformation of large numbers of individuals (i.e., the wellness industry) does not translate into the transformation of our communities. And yet everything around us is underlying our interdependence, from infectious disease to inequality to climate change. For us to survive and thrive, healing must prioritize community. It must center the most vulnerable among us to ensure that all are included and no one is left behind. Understanding ourselves in relationship to one another—and repairing the bonds that have been broken—is critical to our future. Healing is only possible when it is whole.

In many ways, we've mistaken the concept of community for lifestyle. Just because you practice yoga with someone every week, wear similar clothes, and chant mantras together doesn't mean you're committed to

149

their liberation and well-being. Lifestyle enthusiasts express their identity through shared consumption and leisure activities, whereas individuals in community express their identity in relationship to mutual and collective responsibility. While true wellness is rooted in interdependence, the modern manifestation of wellness has emphasized sameness and separation. It has driven relentless seeking at the expense of relationship and cooperation. And it leaves us perpetually longing for the gratification that only comes through knowing oneself in relationship.*

Because we live in a toxic world shaped by legacies of separation, scarcity, and supremacy, we must first recognize the ways we are internalizing and acting out those dynamics with one another. That's why Grace Lee Boggs says, "In order to change/transform the world, [we] must change/transform [our] selves."[38] From that place, we can organize our lives and relationships around our values. And we do it every single day. That is how we build community. By connecting through shared values and practice and building a capacity to be in the "principled struggle" together across lines of difference and conflict. In the words of adrienne maree brown, principled struggle is "when we are struggling for the sake of something larger than ourselves and are honest and direct with one another while holding compassion."[39] Being both critical and compassionate is necessary for the growth of our communities and country. It is how we ask hard questions that challenge us to do better, to be more accountable, and to build the more beautiful world that we all deserve.

The essential challenge of this moment is to transform the isolation and self-interest within dominant culture into connectedness and caring for the whole. A community's ability to thrive is dependent on the quality of relationships. We must attend to how we act and value our interdependence and sense of belonging. We must pay attention to how we extend hospitality, tend to the gaps, and hold one another accountable. Our lives have taught us the power of connecting with and across difference, not in spite of difference. Once we realize we belong to each other, we get to reckon with the fact that each of us is participating in creating this world and therefore

---

* In *Community: The Structure of Belonging at Work*, author Peter Block offers best practices to combat isolation and individualism and build authentic community.

must be a part of healing it. Restoring community is essential to healing the past and creating possibilities for the future we all belong to.

Restoring community is not just about bringing people together, it's about creating the conditions for holding change and possibility. According to one of the principles of *Emergent Strategy*, a book by adrienne maree brown, our work is to find the "conversation in the room that only these people at this moment can have."[40] The right conversations reveal our interconnection, unleash our aliveness, and open us up to healing and possibility. To do that we must build containers that can hold all of us in our truth, complexity, and longing for collective well-being—spaces where we can practice creating a counterculture to the one we have inherited that helps us build new skills and capacities for being together. The practice of how we be together is how we stay present in the face of discomfort, how we hold one another in both our brokenness and our beauty, how we listen for understanding, and how we have conversations about things that matter, even when it's hard.

Social fabric is sewn one relationship at a time. It is how we build trust with one another in big and small ways. It is the courageous conversations that reveal the truth of who we are and who we are to each other. And it is the actions we take for the well-being of everyone. Community is an invitation to know ourselves in relationship with everyone and everything around us. It's where we practice showing up in our truth and being accountable to the whole. This means asking who needs to be in the room and which conversation needs to happen so that we can build deep threads of trust, relationship, and accountability that move us forward.* Rev. Dr. Martin Luther King Jr. spoke to this when he said that "all life is interrelated" and that all of humanity is "caught in an inescapable network of mutuality, tied in a single garment of destiny. Whatever affects one directly, affects all indirectly. I can never be what I ought to be until you are what you ought to be, and you can never be what you ought to be until I am what I ought to be . . . This is the interrelated structure of reality."[41]

---

* Check out this "How to Have Hard Conversations" action guide focused on centering relationship and community care across lines of difference: www.ctznwell.org/action-guides/how-to-have-hard-conversations.

Solidarity is a recognition of our mutual responsibility. It's not so much a concept as it is a practice. We know solidarity by how we feel. Solidarity is how we cross borders we have not crossed before, how we understand struggles that have not been our own, how we meet people we haven't met. The word has its roots in the Latin word *solidum*, which means "equally responsible for a debt." Solidarity is not just feel-good allyship. It's mutuality that is rooted in our commitment to give something up for the sake of the whole, for the good of the collective. Unlike individualism, which pits us against each other, solidarity understands that we are all needed in the struggle toward liberation and well-being, that what is possible can only be revealed in mutual relationship.

But solidarity is more than "we're all in this together." We're not. The reality of coronavirus revealed our interdependence. But it also laid bare the inequities in our systems that determine who gets to be well, who gets to work from home, who gets access to testing and treatment—and whose lives are disposable, whose bodies are worth risking on the front line, whose work doesn't require protection. It revealed both our shared vulnerability and our desperate attempt at self-preservation. It's solidarity that determines whether we send our kids to school if they're sick, or whether we hoard toilet paper or groceries when there is a perceived lack of access, or whether we wear face masks and get vaccines. But it is also solidarity that determines whether we vote for policies like universal healthcare, paid sick leave, and guaranteed basic income to protect the most vulnerable. It's the understanding that none of us are well unless all of us are well. All of which calls us to widen "the circle of human concern." Instead of turning inward, we can expand outward to include more, to see ourselves in each other, and to imagine systems and structures where everyone belongs.[42]

Becoming our best selves isn't some personal revolution. It is the responsibility we have to each other. It is the kind of self-making and world-making that understands we are inextricably tied and creates the conditions where everyone can thrive together. It is locating ourselves as part of a larger ecosystem, where everyone's unique role and contribution are understood and appreciated. Purpose isn't some individual endeavor; it actualizes each and every one of us as part of something bigger than ourselves. And it affirms that our highest, most realized self is one that is understood in relationship and expressed from love. As professor john a. powell reminds us, "This is a call to enhance love, but not just private love. This is a call to enhance public love—justice. This is a call to intentionally support the creation of structures informed by our sense of social justice and spirituality."[43]

This is a call for beloved community.

COLLECTIVE PRACTICE: HAVE COURAGEOUS CONVERSATIONS

Courageous conversations are a source of great possibility. It is in these exchanges that we get to practice showing up, being seen, learning in public, asking for what we need, doing repair work, and "putting our hearts on the line" (in the words of Teo Drake) for the sake of healing and transformation. But generative conversations don't just happen; they require care and consideration. Here are some key practices for creating the conditions for courageous conversations with people you are most proximal to (these can be family members, circles of friends, neighbors, coworkers, peers in wellness spaces, activist circles).*

- Assumptions: Acknowledging what's in the air by naming assumptions, differences, values, and potential tensions helps reduce fear and manage expectations. When we make the invisible visible, in terms of dominant culture and systems and how they are at work in our relationships,

---

* Some of my favorite groups who are building beloved community around a shared worldview of interdependence and collective care are Resonance Network, Thrive Network East Bay, and The BIG We.

we create more possibilities for how we can navigate these intersections. **Reflect on some of the assumptions and perspectives you bring to your relationships and conversations.**

- Agreements: Agreements are the active inquiry and practice of who we want to be together. Making agreements asks "What will help us be present, show up, and go deeper together? How will we hold conflict and disagreement? What practices are we centering to encourage truth-telling and reduce harm?" Here are some agreements I've found to be helpful in creating a container that can hold the complexity of who we are:

  - Locate yourself (this includes understanding your social location and how that informs how you show up in relationship)

  - Attend to impact (in a culture that prioritizes good intentions, it's essential to understand that intents have impacts, which often get overlooked)

  - Try it on (be open to doing something different, and embrace the discomfort that comes with change)

  - Listen with an open heart (welcome differences and be curious about what you don't understand)

  - Practice mutual care (balancing how you take care of the self *and* how you tend to the needs of the collective)

  Discuss what agreements are needed for people to feel present, seen, and supported.

- Accountability: It's not enough to have agreements. We must also consent to engaging them together and hold ourselves and each other accountable to the culture we are cocreating. Accountability affirms that our individual contributions (words and actions) matter to the whole of our community. **Acknowledge when an agreement has been broken, take responsibility, and move toward repair when possible.**

- Access: Belonging demands that we do our best to create the conditions for all types of bodies and minds. Ask "What does each of us need to be here?" If our unique needs aren't met, it can be difficult to show up for the work. Is there a need for physical or mental supports? Are we speaking the same language? Do we have the same analysis? **Explore the needs of the different people involved and if and how those needs can be met.**

- Boundaries: Given our different social locations, we are impacted by systems of oppression in different ways and, therefore, must attend to our different needs with skill and discernment. **Consider when connecting with people with whom you share a lived experience is needed to reduce harm and attend to our different needs and responsibilities.**

- Generative questions: We seek conversations that build trust, create accountability, and unleash possibilities. Powerful questions are key to bringing about this kind of transformation. These are not questions that have right answers, validate the status quo, or even aim to reform it. They are questions that engage people in owning and cocreating the future we all deserve. Here are some examples of powerful questions:

  - What is the commitment you hold that you brought into this room?

- What is a crossroads you face at this stage of the game?
- What is the story you keep telling about the problems of this community?
- What are the gifts you hold that have not been brought fully into the world?
- What declarations are you prepared to make about the possibilities for the future?[44]

Collaborate on which powerful questions will guide your conversation toward healing and possibility.

CHAPTER 6

Wellness beyond Whiteness

> Two hundred fifty years of slavery. Ninety years of Jim Crow. Sixty years of separate but equal. Thirty-five years of racist housing policy. Until we reckon with our compounding moral debts, America will never be whole.
>
> TA-NEHISI COATES

I didn't grow up wanting to be an activist—I grew up wanting to fit in. As a person with many layers of privilege, I didn't have to fight for my rights or pay attention to injustice; I could just look the other way and mind my business. But on 9/11, that life betrayed me and kicked off a long journey of unraveling and becoming. No longer could I simply exist for the well-being of me. I realized I was a part of something bigger than myself and needed to show up for it.

Activism gave me something to do with my privilege and the guilt that came with grappling with it. I knew there was work to be done and that I had something to contribute. I could pay it forward and use my privilege for good. At first I awkwardly fumbled around trying to find my place. I organized fundraisers, educated my yoga students on critical issues, joined direct actions, supported solidarity campaigns. I read books, attended trainings, used woke language, posted memes, and proclaimed myself an ally. I wanted to help. I wanted to do better. I wanted to be good.

In 2012 I joined a group of inspired yogis on a service trip to South Africa. We had raised over $500,000 for local projects and, in turn, got to visit and volunteer. Throughout our time in Cape Town, we learned from local leaders, we built a library, we volunteered at an orphanage, we taught children yoga. We listened, we learned, and then we left. Upon our return home, I posted pictures from our visit. The captions accompanying my pictures were about how much volunteering had taught me and how blessed and transformed I was by the experience. What followed was an avalanche of praise and validation for how selfless and inspiring I was. But was I really? There is no doubt that I was changed by that work. What I witnessed and learned in South Africa was one of the most powerful experiences of my life. I wanted to be proud of the work we did there. I wanted to believe we helped each other. But what if my "good intentions" benefited me more than the projects and people we were serving? Or worse, what if they didn't do good at all?

Well-Meaning White People

My trip to South Africa echoed a long history of white people working out their greed, their guilt, or their good intentions on the lives of people of color around the world. From colonization to missionary work to transracial adoption to foreign policy, the legacy of the white savior is alive and well. It assumes that countries in the Global South desperately need industrialized countries such as the United States to save them, that white Westerners have the right answers, the best expertise, the appropriate resources. It's Christian missionaries and the Peace Corps, but it's also wellness influencers and thought leaders who believe they must be a "voice for the voiceless." But no one is voiceless; they're just unheard, and we're not listening.

In *Me and White Supremacy*, Layla Saad defines white saviorism as "the belief that people with white privilege, who see themselves as superior in capability and intelligence, have an obligation to 'save' [Black, Indigenous, and People of Color] from their supposed inferiority and helplessness."[1] White saviorism looks like volunteers doing work that can be done by local people; it looks like illegitimate international adoptions and "voluntourists" exploiting people (often kids) for feel-good acts of service or, worse, "poverty porn" that exploits children for selfies and social media attention. To justify this, people like me have to buy into the story that countries in the Global South are poor, broken, and hopeless until the white person— the missionary, the philanthropist, the tourist, the military general, the compassionate yogi—comes to fix them. We have to *believe* that they need us. That we white Westerners have it all figured out. That we have what they need. That we are the ones they've been waiting for.

And it's no wonder. White saviorism is center stage throughout mainstream culture, from schools to news media to Hollywood. In blockbuster films like *The Help, The Green Book, Dances with Wolves, The Last Samurai,* and many others, white people are central to the plot of saving people of color, with no mention of the irony that they are the reason people of color are suffering. Still, Hollywood fetishizes these well-intentioned characters, centering white do-gooding while marginalizing the role of people of color in their own liberation and making millions along the way. In education, Eurocentric curricula paint colonialism as discovery and colonists as saviors—reinforcing the idea that white Westerners are the heroes of our past and, therefore, most qualified to solve other people's problems. White kids grow up thinking that white people are exceptional and entitled to "help" others without considering that other people may not need or want their help at all.

Which leads us to foreign policy. Under the banner of humanitarian aid and intervention, the US has historically pillaged countries in the Global South for labor, resources, and military control—only to return later and "save them" after a disaster. Central to this strategy is US exceptionalism, the idea that Americans are exemplary and therefore uniquely qualified to fix other countries' problems, resolve conflicts that we don't understand, and export our toxic ideals (and control). We are so quick to assume our place in "helping the less fortunate" that we fail to acknowledge the role Western imperialism has played in causing the harm in the first place. It is a vicious cycle of cause and effect that ultimately comes back around.

And that leaves white people like me assuming we know what's best. We exclude the voices, experiences, and wisdom of those who are closest to the problem. We force assistance and declare war on other people's behalf. We rob people of their agency, perpetuating narratives of helplessness. And we exploit real people for personal sentiment. When I think back to my time in South Africa, I recall horrific behaviors that anywhere else would be considered completely inappropriate, like picking up and petting children, taking pictures of people like props, and assuming our beliefs, opinions, and ways of being were essential to these people with whom we had no trust or relationship. All of this for the glory of being the hero or, worse, working out our own shame. I later came to understand that I wasn't there for them. I was there for me.

Nigerian American writer Teju Cole says: "Africa has provided a space onto which white egos can conveniently be projected. It is a liberated space in which the usual rules do not apply: A nobody from America or Europe can go to Africa and become a godlike savior, or at the very least, have his or her emotional needs satisfied. Many have done it under the banner of 'making a difference.'"[2] All of which equates to what he calls the White Savior Industrial Complex—an entire industry of tourism, volunteerism, trade, charity, and wellness—that not only profits from but also allows white people to work out their desire to be good on "poor" people of color with no mind to their impact.*

When I went to South Africa, I thought I was making a difference, but it was, at best, a Band-Aid on the gaping wound of colonization and imperialism and, at worst, part of a larger vicious cycle that keeps oppressive

---

* Teju Cole's "White Savior Industrial Complex" is essential reading on the dangers of white saviorism: www.theatlantic.com/international/archive/2012/03/the-white-savior-industrial-complex/254843/.

systems in place. The consequences of these systems are so pervasive and traumatic that they cannot be solved by building a school or sponsoring a child. Well-meaning white people like me need to stop "medicating" ourselves with good intentions and start treating the deeper disease. While the influx of activism and social do-gooding looks good on the surface, there is danger in well-meaning work that doesn't address structural inequities and take into consideration the needs, expertise, and cultural context of people being "helped." White saviorism only serves to keep oppressive systems in place.

We don't need another hero. We need justice.

The Master's House

Growing up, I always felt power was elusive, even while I was striving to get closer to it, to become more "perfect," to earn my place in society. As a woman in a man's world, I understood the toxic consequences of power, sometimes violently. But outside of feeling powerless, I never understood the ways in which I was powerful. Even as a nonprofit executive, I was unaware of the ways I guarded the gate, making decisions about who was included or how to distribute grants and scholarships or what to allocate funds to. I assumed that my good intentions were enough to justify my decisions, regardless of the impacts. But refusing to see how power is at work is the very thing that makes it dangerous and keeps it going.

The desire to be good—whether in the eyes of God, or under the banner of meritocracy, or due to social pressure to be perfect—often has more to do with serving ourselves than the people we are trying to serve. In *Winners Take All: The Elite Charade of Changing the World*, Anand Giridharadas posits that the leaders who are trying to help others while also helping themselves are part of the problem. He calls it the "do well by doing good" paradigm, where do-gooders shore up their position through the power of sponsoring, innovating, and controlling change.[3] It is the trend of social impact investing, tech innovators, conscious capitalists, and wealthy foundations who want to change the world. But Giridharadas argues that people in power aren't just looking to make a difference, they're looking for a win-win. Win-win sounds good in theory. Its idea of "a rising tide lifts all boats" is synonymous with trickle-down economics. But self-interest rarely trickles down.

And where have good intentions gone more unchecked than in philanthropy, where wealthy do-gooders make decisions for communities they do not come from, may not understand, and rarely interact with?[4] Dr. Martin Luther King Jr. said, "Philanthropy is commendable, but it must not cause the philanthropist to overlook the circumstances of economic justice which make philanthropy necessary."[5] He's speaking to the difference between charity and justice. While charity is about helping those in need, justice is about changing the conditions that caused the need in the first place. I'm not saying that donating money is all bad. In fact, the redistribution of wealth through philanthropy has accomplished great things. But charity often treats the symptoms while ignoring the root causes and realities that created the problem and the forces that continue to perpetuate it (of which charity is one). In giving generously, do-gooders often get to feel and look good without ever being accountable for their culpability or complicity in injustice. Not to mention, we wouldn't need philanthropic giving to supplement inadequate social systems if individuals and corporations weren't allowed to amass so much power and wealth in the first place.

Oscar Wilde alluded to this when he said that often "the people who do most harm are the people who try to do most good."[6] We glorify the good deeds of a few (philanthropic funding, in-kind gifts) over fighting for the goodness of all (universal access, redistribution of wealth, living wage). This is especially true among wellness companies that claim to be "conscious," only so far as it does not impact their bottom line. Take Whole Foods, for example, whose founder proclaims the idea of "conscious capitalism" while supporting tax breaks for the rich and calling the Affordable Care Act "fascism."[7] Or Mark Zuckerberg, Elon Musk, and Jeff Bezos, whose companies avoid paying taxes, fight government regulations, and deny their workers vital benefits and a living wage.[8] Elite change-makers insist on *Lean In* circles for women instead of funding paid family leave. They make generous donations for disaster relief and cancer research but refuse to pay their workers hazard pay and sick leave.

They build charter schools but are unwilling to challenge a rigged education system that is designed to favor white elites (by tying school funding to property taxes). Not only does this kind of "generosity" fail to make us better, but it serves to keep inequality intact.

Audre Lorde warned against this when she said that "the master's tools will never dismantle the master's house. They may allow us temporarily to beat him at his own game, but they will never enable us to bring about genuine change."[9] She spoke these words in 1979 on a panel called "The Personal Is Political" to point out the failures of white feminism in defeating white patriarchy.* Power and change are intimately connected. Power is defined as one's ability to influence and define reality for ourselves and others, in ways that are both visible and hidden. It often manifests as influence, access to resources, rules and regulations, control over bodies and choices, decision-making, and the ability to shape narratives and culture. Power is neither good nor bad, but it does have consequences. For example, the power that marginalized people experience is often "power over"—the power that people and institutions have over their lives, their children, their mobility, their access to basic needs, and their self-determination—whereas the dominant group has the power (through access and decision-making) to not only create their own reality but create the reality of others.

To understand how power works, we must ask who benefits (via access, rights, wealth, well-being), who governs (via representation and ability to shape policy), and who wins (via decision-making power). And in America, those in power are unmistakable—white people make up 90 percent of elected officials, 96 percent of senior leadership roles in US companies, 80 percent of Congress, 80 percent of federal judges, 65 percent of police officers, 94 percent of Fortune 500 CEOs, 80 percent of board seats, and 78 percent of school administrators. And there is no greater indicator of power than those who occupy the top 1 percent in America, controlling more than 30 percent of all wealth in the country, 96 percent of whom are white and male.[10] Nearly all of

---

* Dig deeper into the dangers of white feminism with *Hood Feminism: Notes from the Women That a Movement Forgot* by Mikki Kendall and *White Tears, Brown Scars: How White Feminism Betrays Women of Color* by Ruby Hamad.

the most powerful people in the United States—those who control our institutions, our economies, and our cultural realities—are white. And the rest of us are the gatekeepers who "guard the gate" of power, determining who, when, and how to open and close the door of access and advantage that impacts other people's lives and well-being. All of which keeps us stuck in the cycle of social control and supremacy.

The Color of Supremacy

I grew up in a white town with white friends. I went to a white school and played white sports and had white boyfriends. In university, I went to white bars with white students. Afterward I got a white job working with white coworkers making a white salary. When I married a white guy, all the people at my wedding were white. And then I became another white yoga teacher doing white yoga in the white wellness industry. But if you had asked me if I knew I was white, if I was aware of my racial identity and all the advantages it affords me, I would have said, "No! That's just how it is." But "how it is" in America—how it has always been—is a deeply racialized world invented to determine who gets to be well and who doesn't.

James Baldwin said, "No one was white before he/she came to America."[11] Before that, people were from the lands upon which they were born and raised. They saw themselves as Irish or Yoruba or German or Guarani. But as America came into being, the legal designation of white became necessary to determine who fits where in the hierarchy. My own ancestors existed for many years as Irish and Italian before they were reimagined as "white." The social and legal construction of race justified the dominance of the people who came to be known as white.[12] "White people" were invented as a structure of social control that used racist policies and privileges to protect the interest of the ruling class.* Isabel Wilkerson, author of *Caste: The Origins of Our Discontents*, calls it "America's enduring caste system."[13]

---

* For more on the construction of whiteness, check out Noel Ignatiev's *How the Irish Became White* and *The Invention of White Race: Racial Oppression and Social Control* by Theodore Allen.

Caste is a deeply entrenched yet artificial structure of categorizing people, and race is fundamental to underpinning that structure. When assigning race, we're not just recognizing difference, we're giving significance and attributing assumptions, values, and rank to particular groups of people. Race is the visible indicator of our place in the hierarchy of human value—pointing to things like how we are treated by doctors, or whether we will live adjacent to a toxic waste plant, or if we will be considered for the promotion, or how likely we are to be pulled over and harmed by law enforcement. Any system that ranks human value is not natural, but it is very much alive.*

It's tempting to assume that race was constructed because of ignorance and hate, but according to author and historian Ibram X. Kendi, we have cause and effect backward. Kendi asserts that race and racist policies were actually constructed because of self-interest—then racist policies led to racist ideas, which in turn led to ignorance and hate. These roots can be traced back to the feudalism of medieval Europe, when the Irish, Jews, Romans, and others deemed inferior were victims of invasion, dispossession, and violence.[14] Exploitation was the project of imperialism and colonialism, and racist ideas were used to justify the accumulation of land, wealth, and power by elites.[15] It is the paradox that we live with today: a nation founded on ideals of freedom and independence ended up depending on, defending, and protecting the oppression of entire peoples for the privilege of another.† But none of us is free inside this system.

Justifying the spoils and supremacy of whiteness required making up stories that dehumanized people. Native people were "savages" and Black people were "animals," and it was the white man's job to "save" them for

---

* These podcasts are essential listening on the history and invention of race: *1619* and *Seeing White*.

† For more on racial capitalism check out *Change Everything: Racial Capitalism and the Case for Abolition* by Ruth Wilson Gilmore, *Black Marxism: The Making of the Black Radical Tradition* by Cedric Robinson, and "Understanding and Organizing to End Racial Capitalism" by SURJ featuring Robin D. G. Kelley: www.surj.org/understanding-and-organizing-to-end-racial-capitalism-with-dr-robin-dg-kelley/.

their own good. The racial order would become ingrained in law, science, religion, and culture, further entrenching the story. As times changed, so would racism, mutating and morphing from slavery to Jim Crow to mass incarceration, all to accommodate white power and privilege.[16] The staying power of this ideology lives on in us today. As Wilkerson notes, "To dehumanize another human being is not merely to declare that someone is not human, and it does not happen by accident. It is a process, a programming. It takes energy and reinforcement to deny what is self-evident in another member of one's own species."[17]

Racism operates on us mentally, emotionally, physically, and spiritually. Throughout our lives, we absorb racist cultural messages that present white people as whole human beings while dehumanizing Blackness, invisibilizing Indigenous people, and regarding everyone who isn't white as inferior. White people, consciously and unconsciously, internalize messages of superiority—of being normal, qualified, objective, entitled, justified, and innocent. The inverse is a narrative of inferiority among people of color, who internalize self-doubt, self-hate, powerlessness, a limited sense of potential, and hopelessness. These ideas become deep-seated in our subconscious and expressed through our behaviors. Of course, this is not *who we are* but it is what we are taught by dominant culture. Through socialization, we are trained to play the roles that we are assigned.

Growing up in America demanded that I learn how to be white. It said I had to be perfect, and yet I was never good enough. It said that I had a right to comfort, and when I'm not comfortable, something is wrong and someone is to blame. It said I was innocent and worthy of protection. It said that I could be anything I wanted to be and I was welcome everywhere. It said to be afraid and never admit it. It said that I should help those less fortunate even if they don't want my help. It encouraged me to be good and to prove I am better than others. Privilege only reinforced this ideology, granting me assumed credibility and leadership, the freedom to move as I desired, unquestioned access to rooms and spaces, a right to comfort, and more. I was forever surrounded by an onslaught of positive messages saying that it was better to be white, that white people were normal, deserving, justified, and innocent . . . until I believed it. Believing these things was the price of belonging to a white world—and to the wellness world.*

Wellness is just one more invitation to climb the ladder. To be well and fit and mindful is the symbol of our status. In *The Sum of Small Things: A Theory of the Aspirational Class*, Elizabeth Currid-Halkett talks about how many elites now express their position not by purchasing expensive flashy things but by signaling their superiority through buying organic products, driving hybrid cars, and meditating religiously.[18] These enthusiasts can't resist an opportunity to moralize and proselytize (and troll) the superior benefits of wellness embodied in the image of the superior white body. Brands like Bulletproof and Goop promise to make you not just superior but superhuman. And while white people are celebrated for biohacking and cold plunges, people of color are stigmatized, pathologized, and punished for not living up to the expectation of white wellness.

But this isn't just about whether racism exists in the wellness industry; it's about how wellness actually reinforces racism. From cultural appropriation to whitewashed media and product development to luxury pricing, wellness isn't a victim of white supremacy, it's a perpetrator. Instead of pointing toward our true nature, wellness encourages us to strive for more and climb the ladder. It says that we are not enough unless we are at the top. But the top is an impossible destination that most of us will never reach, no matter how hard we try. Which is exactly what keeps the system going. The ladder of racial hierarchy is only real because we keep trying to climb it.[19] For racial order to exist, Americans had to invent it (race), defend it (Jim Crow), and then maintain it (policing).

---

* Tema Okun, in collaboration with her late colleague and mentor Kenneth Jones, wrote an article in 1999 on the characteristics of white supremacy to better understand the "water" we are swimming in, so that we may more skillfully navigate the culture and choose to create something new. She has since revised and updated the content at www.whitesupremacyculture.info /characteristics.html.

Policing Bodies

I remember teaching a yoga class in 2014 around the time of Eric Garner's murder. At the beginning of class, as I always do, I invited people to breathe freely. And I was struck by how utterly privileged that was in the context of Garner's brutal murder. His words "I can't breathe" would be echoed years later by George Floyd and at least seventy other Black men who were unjustly killed by law enforcement after saying those words.[20] This refrain has been invoked again and again in the activism and advocacy of the Black Lives Matter movement as a reminder of what we are fighting for. Michelle Cassandra Johnson testifies to this in her book *Skill in Action* when she says, "White supremacy takes my breath away."[21] It is the breath denied by a knee on one's neck. It is the breath compromised by asthma due to environmental racism. It is the breath taken away by COVID-19 at more than double the rate of white people.[22] It is the breath held in response to microaggressions and macroviolence. And it is the breath policed and silenced to uphold the system in all its mutations.

The racial caste system only works when everyone stays in their place. That's where policing comes in. From its origins as slave patrols, policing has served as a violent arm of the racist caste system by protecting the interests of white elites and controlling people of color—particularly Black people—through everyday surveillance, intimidation, arrests, and incarceration. Today, getting killed by the police is a leading cause of death for young Black men.[23] And one out of every four will end up in the prison system.* But state-sanctioned surveillance and control extends well beyond law enforcement. Take the child welfare system, which more accurately should be called the "family regulation system," in how it regulates millions of marginalized people through "wellness checks," investigations, and the forced removal of children, most of which don't stem from bad parenting but from the consequences of poverty.[24] Or consider the militarization of schools, wherein Black kids are suspended and expelled at three times the rate of white kids.[25] (And

---

* Learn more about the legacy of policing and mass incarceration with *Freedom Is a Constant Struggle* by Angela Davis, *The New Jim Crow* by Michelle Alexander, and *Invisible No More: Police Violence against Black Women and Women of Color* by Andrea Ritchie.

they are three times more likely to end up in the juvenile system.*) Or take the racist immigration policies that have detained, deported, separated, and destroyed countless immigrant families. Social control poisons our public institutions and makes them weapons of the state, intended to support racial order, not public well-being.

But policing isn't only expressed through the state. It is also enforced through culture. This informal form of social control follows a set of rules and standards that keeps people bound to playing our roles and upholding the social order. It includes symbolic policing that governs how people of color are allowed to be, where they are allowed to go, what decisions they're allowed to make. For example, professionalism in the workplace privileges white cultural norms and demands that people of color code-switch to keep up. It operates according to a specific set of attributes designed to police the status quo and uphold white capitalism. According to social justice trainer and facilitator Tema Okun, the attributes of white supremacy culture are difficult to identify because they operate in the backdrop as norms and standards without being recognized, named, or chosen. Norms like perfectionism, paternalism, either/or thinking, power hoarding, valuing quantity over quality, and individualism are not only prevalent in our culture, they're enforced. You're either playing by the rules or you're paying the consequences.[26]

Which brings us to how we police each other. Dr. King spoke of this in "Letter from a Birmingham Jail" when he said, "I have been gravely disappointed with the white moderate . . . who is more devoted to 'order' than to justice; who prefers a negative peace which is the absence of tension to a positive peace which is the presence of justice; who constantly says: 'I agree with you in the goal you seek, but I cannot agree with your methods of direct action.'"[27] In response to facts and uncomfortable truths, those of us who are white will often do whatever is possible to protect our comfort in a situation where white supremacy is being challenged. These

---

* Bettina Love explores the "educational survival complex" and the institutional barriers that are in the way of Black and Brown students' success and what we can do about it in *We Want to Do More Than Survive: Abolitionist Teaching and the Pursuit of Educational Freedom.*

microaggressions include criticizing how people of color engage in their own liberation or even talk about their own lived experience. It is all of the ways white people defend their comfort and innocence in order to maintain control.

As a white woman, I've become painfully aware of how white women's perceived innocence has been a tool to maintain white supremacy for centuries—particularly when it comes to policing Black men. Whether white women are calling the police on Black men who are birdwatching, or going for a jog, or simply entering their own apartment, they are following in an unspeakably violent and centuries-long tradition of white women whose accusations (real or false) against Black men resulted in mob violence and lynchings. But as Stephanie Jones-Rogers writes in her book *They Were Her Property: White Women as Slave Owners in the American South*, it's no shock the way that some white women respond to interactions with Black people today because white women were, in fact, deeply invested and engaged in the system of slavery that benefited them in every way it benefited white men.[28] To this day white women are quick to assume authority to surveil, suspect, accuse, and remove Black people from their lives. And it works. More often than not, Black "suspects" are asked to leave, apprehended, or worse. Meanwhile, white women can count on being given the benefit of the doubt, being assumed to be innocent, and being trusted as telling the truth and acting in the best interest of white people regardless of the circumstances.

Wellness, an industry and culture dominated by white women, is particularly thorough in how it enforces this social order. Because policing isn't just about restricting other people's freedom; it's also about entitlement and social control. Under the guise of love and light and pastel hues is a whitewashed culture that thrives off shaming bodies, exploiting marginalized people, and centering whiteness. This manifestation of policing looks like stealing and appropriating Indigenous culture, whitewashing it, and profiting from it. It is white ownership that creates the policies that govern price of entry, accessibility, ethics, safety, leadership, and programming. It is tokenizing and exploiting Black and Brown bodies for the optics of diversity. And it is bypassing and shutting down conversations about race and oppression, avoiding social justice issues to "keep the peace," and demanding "positive vibes only." Tone policing in this way is an extension of the violence practiced against Black people, Indigenous folks, and other people of color every day. It silences marginalized voices by calling out the tone of the message over the content of the message. Tone policing is demanding that conversations about trauma and harm be civil and calm and nice. It is avoiding accountability and repair. And it is placing white comfort above the well-being of people of color.

All of which feeds into a carceral culture that becomes ingrained in our consciousness.* Carceral logics encourage us to blame the problem on the individual when harm occurs and then isolate, punish, and often stigmatize that individual and the community they are a part of. It is done in overt ways by the state and criminal system, but also more subtle indirect ways that normalize punitive responses and celebrate redemptive violence, like when a child misbehaves in school and we suspend (exclude) them from the classroom, or when a colleague says something that makes us uncomfortable and we publicly shame them, or when we report neighbors for things we don't agree with and risk their eviction, or when we humiliate people on social media and encourage others to cancel them. These examples contribute to a culture that normalizes punishment and isolation as a response to social problems. Rather than looking at root causes and trying to understand why a problem emerged in the first place, we default to blame, retaliation, and punishment. We respond by distancing ourselves, removing people, and marking them as different from the rest of us.[29]

Policing and carceral logic are in all of us who steeped in the system of racism and white supremacy. And while we occupy different locations, everybody is situated inside this system. It is how we control others from a position of power, but it is also how we are controlled. That's because

---

* The term *carceral* refers to the variety of ways our bodies, minds, and actions have been shaped by the ideas and practices of policing and imprisonment.

policing demands obedience and submission in order to function. In *Radical Dharma*, Rev. angel Kyodo williams writes:

> *That mandate is to control Black bodies.*
>
> *The need is to have the constant specter of the other.*
>
> *When the other exists, it strengthens your need to belong.*
>
> *Your belonging is necessary for compliance.*
>
> *Your compliance maintains the system.*
>
> *You are policed too.*
>
> *You are policed by your need for belonging.*
>
> *Your need for belonging requires control of the other.*
>
> *... Or at least the illusion of it.*
>
> *You are policed through the control of my body.*
>
> *You are policed too.*[30]

None of us is truly free in a culture of policing. "The reality of American freedom is that it requires that many of us remain captive to preserve the illusion of freedom for all," says Dr. Jasmine Syedullah.[31] She's speaking to how we've had to be judge and jury to each other for not living up to the American ideal—for not being white enough, for not being American enough, for not being independent enough, and so on. Understanding the cost of this mindset is essential to getting free from it.

The Cost of Whiteness

"I can't possibly be racist! I meditate!" Back in the day, this was my mantra and the mantra of so many who equate "goodness" with not-racist. Like many, I grew up believing that white supremacy was an extreme behavior done by some bad people other than myself. I'd think of the KKK or Nazis, but never me, never my people. I wasn't perfect, but I was "good." Good was my front-and-center innocent intentions regardless of the impacts. And it was my performance of niceness intended to drown out conflict and discomfort. All of this of course only served to protect one thing: my precious ego. Individualism had me believing that I could step outside of racism and be pure—that I could meditate and escape to ashrams and cleanse the toxicity with juice fasts and plant medicines. So I would hide. I would pretend to be OK. I would act like I knew better. I would point the finger. I would take the high road. All to escape the possibility that I might not be good or perfect or right. But the idea that any of us can be exempt from white supremacy and the forces of socialization is exactly what allows white supremacy to persist and destroy.

One of the great misperceptions that keeps white supremacy alive is the belief that white supremacy is about bad people doing bad things. But the overt racism of people like Donald Trump and the Proud Boys is simply its most visible product. Rather, "white supremacy is not a shark, it is the water," says spoken-word poet Guante.[32] The water—of white supremacy and privilege—is the many systems that determine our well-being: healthcare, housing, economy, education. But it is also the centuries of systemic disadvantage, discrimination, and violence that people of color have faced—and continue to face today. This water is difficult to see, particularly for white people, precisely because white people are swimming in it, immersed in it, and benefiting from it. Which effectively keeps white supremacy in power: its ability to remain invisible and elusive.

From this system stems whiteness—a dominant cultural space constructed with the purpose of keeping white people in the center and others on the margin. Whiteness isn't a "thing"; it is not biological, geographical, or cultural. Its power is manifested through social, political, and cultural behavior with very real, tangible, and violent effects. Under the cover of white privilege, those of us who are white are not directly confronted with everyday effects of racism, which can cause us to "not see color" or to overlook our own white racial status. I didn't grow up knowing I was white or as raced as any person of color, and not knowing was how I avoided the uncomfortable reality that the system is rigged for white people like me. But colorblindness has long been a tool used to maintain, not change, power structures. Decades after Jim Crow was abolished, Americans continue to live deeply segregated lives, which makes it possible for white people to live, grow, and die without ever having interracial connection. The coveted "good schools" and "safe neighborhoods" that I grew up in are simply code for *white* and *better*. Individualism and meritocracy insulate those of us who are white from racial literacy, convincing us that our achievements are the result of our hard work alone, unaided by racial advantages. All of this sets us up to uphold the horrors of systemic racism and ignore the consequences.

The cost of not being white in this society is well documented. People of color—particularly Black Americans and Indigenous people—have significantly lower income and wealth, higher levels of poverty and exposure to environmental toxins, greater health comorbidities, and shorter lifespans compared to white people. But the impact on people of color goes well beyond statistics. It is the acute theft of labor that has created catastrophic material inequality, and it is the countless lives lost to white greed. It is the transhistorical trauma passed down through generations. It is the relentless political disenfranchisement and disempowerment that is embedded in the nation's founding. It is impossible to calculate exactly what America owes to Black Americans, Indigenous Peoples, and other people of color for their contributions to this country and the history of harm they endured. Eula Biss calls it white debt, "reckoning with what is owed—and what can never be repaid—for racial privilege."[33]

But the impacts of racism land differently on (and in) bodies. To understand whiteness is to confront anti-Blackness and the real life-or-death consequences related to the darkness of one's skin. Anti-Blackness represents the unique position Black people were assigned at the bottom of the hierarchy of bodies and the policies, past and present, that exist to keep Black people oppressed while upholding whiteness. The unjust legacies of slavery and violence rooted in anti-Black racism date back more than 400 years and persist to this day through structural and systemic inequalities in education, economic opportunity, policing, health care, housing, criminal justice, and more. In contrast with the way Black people have been racialized as property (and later criminals), Indigenous Peoples have been systemically erased through displacement and removal, forced assimilation, and attempted genocide. Today Indigenous people experience the highest rates of systemic racism in the United States: they are more likely to be killed by police than any other race, Native women are 2.5 times more likely than women of any other racial group to be raped or sexually harassed, Native youth have the lowest graduation rates, and Native Americans have the highest poverty rates and the lowest life expectancy of all racial groups.[34]

There was a saying in the 1960s: "If you're white, you're all right. If you're black, stay back. If you're brown, stick around."[35] The idea was that the country would accept non-Black people into society . . . eventually. But the truth is that anyone in the middle of the racial hierarchy can only ever experience conditional privilege—benefits that can be revoked at any time. Coronavirus revealed how quickly the "model minority" stereotype among Asian Americans can shift to "yellow peril" in white supremacy culture.[36] Arab Americans experienced similar scapegoating in the aftermath of 9/11, resulting in increased surveillance, immigration restrictions, and harmful stereotypes.[37] Latinx people are stereotyped as being "illegal" and have long been othered and accused of taking white jobs and status, resulting in a legacy of being undocumented, unprotected, and underpaid.[38] All the while, white supremacy divides communities of color through tools like colorism, which pits lighter-skinned people against those with darker complexions to distract from the real oppression: white supremacy.*

Meanwhile, white supremacy costs all of us. Racism is the common denominator for some of the biggest threats to our collective well-being and survival, such as climate change, inequality, and threats to democracy. And while white people are manipulated by white cultural politics, the wealthy and powerful get a bigger piece of the pie. The fallout of this racial bargain is the slow and persistent erosion of economic and social security that has left white people scrambling for ground. In fact, the majority of Americans making under $15 an hour are white, as are the majority of people without health insurance.[39] And yet those of us who are white often collude with disempowerment. A majority of white voters in this country have time and time again chosen to vote for the preservation of white supremacy over

---

* To truly understand how different groups have been racialized and impacted by the culture and system of white supremacy, it is best to listen directly to their voices and stories and follow their lead. Please see "Keep Going" at the back of the book for resources.

their own physical and economic well-being. These are in no way comparable to the substantive economic, political, and social costs that people of
color experience due to everyday racism. But they are consequences, nonetheless, that have both material and psycho-spiritual costs to white people's
individual and collective well-being.

The accumulation of harm passed down through generations lives
on in white people today. The white body has been shaped by trauma—
inherited and reinforced by repeated exposure to the inhumanity of colonization and white supremacy. White settlers brought to the American col-
onies a great deal of unresolved trauma from the impoverished and violent
conditions of the Middle Ages. Upon arrival, many traded in their cultural
origins to assimilate and belong in white America, leaving them grasping
for meaning and membership in a young and wounded world. In my own
exploration of who and where I come from, I've discovered a number of
severed lines and lineages. Family histories were abandoned in order to
assimilate into the "security" of white supremacy. They are my lost ancestors: witches run out of Salem, Jews converted to a more socially acceptable
Catholicism, Italian immigrants who hustled to prove themselves worthy
of whiteness. We know the rest. Hurt people hurt people. And until those
of us who are white reckon with the wound that lies underneath the
shield of whiteness—our racialized trauma, our unconscious biases, our
internalized superiority, our defensive behaviors—we will never be well.

Maintaining the myth of whiteness requires a level of disownment and
dissociation that is toxic to the white body. The cost to avoiding the pain
of our own racism is that we've become disembodied, unable to feel, and
apathetic in the face of horrific suffering. In exchange for the privileges of
white supremacy, white people have had to fear, disown, humiliate, ignore,
dehumanize, murder, incarcerate, and segregate ourselves from the majority of humanity. White people may have physical health advantages by not
being subject to the stressors of systemic racism, but even despite our racial
privilege, data suggests that white people are experiencing disproportionate psychiatric challenges compared to other groups. Since the mid-1990s,
reports of chronic pain, mental distress, prescription drug addiction, and
suicide have increased significantly in white communities.[40] Deaths of

despair are on the rise due to lack of dignity of work, the humiliation of joblessness, the loss of economic hope, the lack of social belonging.[41] But some believe that these illnesses are a sign of "white rage" turned inward.*

"This problem, which they invented in order to safeguard their purity, has made of them criminals and monsters, and it is destroying them," James Baldwin says. "And this not from anything blacks may or may not be doing but because of the role a guilty and constricted white imagination has assigned to the blacks."[42] For white supremacy to thrive there must always be a subordinate group to oppress. Anyone with a marginalized identity could at any time be castigated from the dominant group and subject to exclusion, exploitation and oppression. White supremacy is a toxin in the American body that is making us all sick. Fostering well-being for ourselves and one another demands that we reckon with our collusion with white supremacy and work toward accountability and repair that affirm all life and ensure everyone is taken care of. Our full humanity can only be realized in full community with other human beings.

---

* Carol Anderson defines "white rage" as the policies that undermine Black achievement and advancement in her book *White Rage: The Unspoken Truth of Our Racial Divide*.

RECOVERY

> If you have come here to help me you are wasting your
> time, but if you have come because your liberation is
> bound up with mine, then let us work together.
>
> ABORIGINAL ACTIVISTS GROUP*

Once I woke up to whiteness, I was determined to be a "good ally." One of the first solidarity initiatives I worked on was Fight for 15, a campaign among fast-food workers to raise the minimum wage to $15 per hour. I was a part of a multiracial working group that had signed on to mobilize the wellness community around a living wage and economic justice. At the time the federal minimum wage was $7.25 (still is), and companies like McDonald's, who employed millions of people around the country, were paying poverty wages and denying workers benefits and the right to unionize (while their CEO took home almost 2000 times that of the average worker). Fast-food companies employ almost 5 million workers in the US, many of whom are women with children.[43]

I threw myself into the work—planning actions, running meetings, making spreadsheets. I was driven to do my part as a privileged person and make an impact. As the event approached, things ramped up and I drove harder. I felt that people weren't pulling their weight and consensus was time consuming, so I took the lead and pushed through. I thought if I did more and gave more I was being a good ally. I noticed tension on the team, but it felt more important to deliver results than to pause and find out what was going on.

When I was confronted by some Black members of the group for taking control and making unilateral decisions, I got defensive. How else were we to meet our deadlines? If I didn't take charge, the work wouldn't get done, and it most definitely wouldn't get done "right." I was just doing what I had

---

* Read about these activists' history and the authorship of this quote in a post by Ricardo Levins Morales on the Northland Poster Collective's blog, via the Internet Archive: https://uniting .church/lilla-watson-let-us-work-together/.

to do to deliver. Making an impact was more important than anything else, right? Wrong. It took me a long time to see the impact of my actions. My so-called allyship was just a cover for maintaining power. I was more committed to being in control and getting shit done than to how people felt in the process. I blamed tight deadlines and righteous action for behaviors that excluded, dismissed, and harmed people I cared about. From perfectionism to power hoarding to a sense of urgency to individualism, I embodied the very weapons that keep white supremacy in place. Because I chose to put my attachment to comfort and control above everyone else's experience, I not only compromised the project, but I lost relationships.

Detoxing from whiteness meant confronting my own addiction to control and power and the behaviors that maintain white supremacy, but it also meant being accountable in relationship to myself and others. It was years before I had the opportunity to apologize to the people I harmed in that experience. By that time my defensiveness had given way to humility and heartbreak, and I owned up to my actions. I realized that if we are not centering care and prioritizing relationships in our activism, then we are not doing the work. There is no righteous cause or goal that justifies causing harm in the process. We must live into what we are trying to create if we want to achieve justice and return to community with one another.

If complicity and coercion are how white supremacy has gone on this long, accountability is how we will dismantle it. Accountability calls us to detox from the culture of whiteness that has upheld and sustained an inhumane system and abolish the idea of supremacy that lives with us all. Owning our part in this mess is how we address internalized oppression and do the work of deconstructing white supremacy within ourselves and one another. But it is also how we come into community and work across lines of difference for collective healing and liberation. There is too much at stake; we will never be whole as a people unless we deal with the wound of white supremacy. In particular, those of us who are white must decide that our humanity is more important than our comfort and privilege, and we must choose life-affirming practices that celebrate everyone's value and wholeness. Only then can we recover what has been lost to whiteness, move into relationships of accountability, and build a wellness beyond whiteness.

Recovering Our Humanity from the Delusion of Whiteness

It took me thirty-plus years of willful negligence before I admitted that I was racist, which prompted a long and painful journey of reckoning with my addiction to whiteness and recovering my humanity. A white friend once said to me, "But how could we have known?" She was referring to how racism has been invisibilized by dominant culture, mass media, and our education system. But how could we have not known? For those of us who have a college education, or have access to books and Google, or have the freedom to travel and move in the world . . . *how could we possibly "not know"?* Or did we know and choose to forget? Knowing means taking responsibility for how we've been complicit, how we've allowed whiteness to reign. Knowing means reckoning with how we've benefited from such a horrific and harmful system. And knowing compels us to do the work.

The politics of dehumanization in America goes back to this country's beginning. While we can't undo the past, we can change the course for our collective future. And that is only possible by detoxing from the ideology of supremacy that dictates that some lives are worth more than others. This toxin has infiltrated every corner of the country, deeming some superior and worthy of resources, validation, opportunity, and protection, while others, those deemed inferior, are simply considered less than, stepped on, used, abused, and exploited for the benefit of those in power. As a white person, I can see myself in this system—all the ways I have been taught to expect special treatment but trained to not see it. To see it would require me to reckon with not just my complicity but the harm that has emanated from my white body in a system that has been designed for me at the expense of others.

Race is embedded in our brains and bodies. It is real-time and also inherited from past generations. It is alive in everything we say and do. And while the impact on people of color is undeniable, little is spoken of the moral injury at the heart of whiteness. At our backs is an elaborate cultural system that was created to justify the slave economy and all that came with it. Everything—laws, religious beliefs, educational systems, and more—had to be organized in such a way as to maintain a particular system of brutality and dehumanization. But it is also who white people had to *be* and what white people had to allow in order to let racism thrive. It's how I spent decades of my life going along to get along, choosing not to see the blatant discrimination and racial violence that was all around, refusing to take responsibility for my complicity.

But it's not as simple as doing nothing. In fact, it takes great effort to pretend white supremacy isn't happening, to avoid responsibility, to blame others for their plight, to deny the truth of who we are and how we got here. Living with the stain of white supremacy requires those of us who are white to lie and cheat, to defend our innocence, and to numb our shame. It's why we fall prey to feel-good antidotes, addictions, and distractions (of which wellness culture is one). But there is no true wellness practice or spiritual path that denies the truth of our suffering or the existence of oppression. To heal from the toxicity of whiteness, we white people must be willing to feel the pain of our own racism.

Disembodiment (through inability to feel, dissociation, defensiveness) is a function of white supremacy. It keeps us shut down and apathetic in the face of so much suffering. But this only serves to keep white supremacy in place. Healing requires us to peel back the layers of conditioning, so that we can process the pain, grief, and longing that we carry with us. The body is the gateway to understanding, navigating, and reconciling our unique role and responsibility in the dynamic system of oppression. It demands to be felt. In the years following my time in the Fight for 15 campaign, I learned that as a white person, if I'm not uncomfortable, I'm not doing the work. I learned that discomfort is simply an indication that I'm doing something unfamiliar. It is a signal that I am feeling my way into new territory, and that's exactly what's needed. Discomfort calls us to dig deep and choose, against all our fears of being bad and wrong and guilty, to learn something new and do something different.

Detoxing from the wound of white supremacy didn't just call me to show up for those who have been harmed or oppressed, it called me to show up for myself. I had to examine my own insecurity and shame and how that manifested into racist behavior.* How my impossible expectations of perfection for myself caused me to project that onto others and punish them for not living up to it. How I chose to protect my precious and fragile self at the expense of other people's well-being. How my need to be seen and validated inspired competition over cooperation. How time and time again I chose to burn myself to the ground to avoid the vulnerability of asking for help. How all of this made me conspirator to whiteness. Any system that perpetuates lack of enoughness isn't just bad for you, it is toxic for everyone else.

Waking up to whiteness required that I do what the 12-step program calls a "fearless and searching moral inventory" of not only how I had been complicit but how I had caused real harm.[44] I spent so much of my life trying to be good and perfect that it was inconceivable (and intolerable) to me that that very behavior might be causing harm to others. But to be born in a white body is to be implicated at birth. Every leg up and advantage I received for being white came at a cost to others. Beyond privilege, I had to reckon with how I had excluded others to guard the gate of white power, how I had exploited and tokenized people of color in my work, how I had been unwilling to cede control and power at the expense of my relationships, how I had prioritized my comfort over others' freedom and expression time and time again, and how I had hurt people that I love to protect my precious white ego. Eventually I realized that what I was losing was so much greater than what I was protecting. Whiteness has cost me relationships and connection, it has cut me off from essential parts of myself and my history, and it has held me back from possibility and limited my imagination. Ultimately whiteness has robbed me of my well-being, because no one is well inside of a system of domination, not even white people. It was connecting to this heartbreak and grieving what has been lost that inspired me to become a traitor to white supremacy and choose something different.

---

* Here are some helpful workbooks and resources on examining white supremacy: *Me and White Supremacy* by Layla Saad, *My Grandmother's Hands* by Resmaa Menakem, *The Racial Healing Handbook* by Anneliese A. Singh, *So You Wanna Talk about Race* by Ijeoma Oluo, *The Inner Work of Healing Racial Justice* by Rhonda Magee, and *Radical Dharma: Talking Race, Love, and Liberation* by Rev. angel Kyodo williams, Lama Rod Owens, and Dr. Jasmine Syedullah.

When I account for the harm I have done, the harm I am a part of, I can begin to heal and repair the relationships that have been broken. When I get curious about how toxic beliefs and behaviors live inside of me, I can approach this work with humility and compassion for myself and everyone else who is trying to unlearn white supremacy and imagine something better. I, like so many, am yearning for a world beyond what whiteness has taught us about who is whole and human and worthy of well-being and who isn't. And that is what accountability is asking us to do: to account for our place in the whole. Practicing accountability is how we come back into community with one another. It doesn't just right wrongs and repair relationships; it reveals the interlocking nature of our oppression and the mutuality of our liberation. While we all occupy different locations in this fucked-up system of oppression, our survival requires all of us to show up in love and accountability for the future that we all deserve.

Which begs the question "What has kept white people engaged in the cycle of oppression for so long?" While many attribute our complicity to what we are trying to avoid or escape, I think it has more to do with what we white people are trying to protect. What is so important to us that we would actively choose a system of advantage that requires the oppression of others? Is it preserving our innocence? Or maintaining our position in society? Or attachment to material wealth? Or protection of our ego? Examining the motivations that lie underneath our collusion is essential to unhooking from them. And then we're left to simply choose. Will we stay attached to the false security of whiteness and the dehumanizing ideology of supremacy despite the costs? Or will we do something different? When we go from believing "that's just the way it is" to believing we can change, when we discover that we are capable of more than oppression and retribution, when we choose life over death, then we will all experience the liberation and well-being we have been longing for.

Sonya Renee Taylor says, "'Who am I outside of what whiteness has assigned me?' is a question that might get us all free."[45] It speaks to both what has been lost and negotiated to whiteness and what is possible beyond a system of domination and superiority. While I never consciously identified with whiteness, it was all I knew. I did not understand how to belong outside of whiteness. I didn't know who I was beyond the roles I had to play and rules I was supposed to follow. And for far too long, I wasn't brave enough to risk my comfort and imagine better. I don't know what lies beyond whiteness, who we will be when we reclaim what has been left behind and choose to show up for the whole of who we are. But I believe it is more.

To betray white supremacy—to return to humanity—is to completely divest from the inhumane belief that some lives are worth more than others and to do everything in our power to dismantle the structures that emerged from it. And from that place, perhaps we can show up more fortified and courageous in what Austin Channing Brown calls the "anti-racism work of becoming better humans for other humans."[46]

White people have traded in humanity in order to fit into a culture of good and greed. And it has taken everything from us—our connectedness, our humanity, our future. Recovering from this wound calls those of us who are white to build a new way of being human with other humans. It must include a historical analysis of how we got here, an understanding of the systems that continue to perpetuate injustice, and a practice that embraces accountability and upholds the dignity and humanity of all people. This cannot be theoretical in nature. It must be an everyday practice that moves us toward wholeness with one another. We must no longer strive to be good; we must strive to be human. Together.

PERSONAL INQUIRY

Reckoning with how whiteness has shaped me requires that I be both critical and compassionate. I find that capacity on my mat when I come up against parts of myself I'm ashamed of. I meet the tough edges and tension with softness. I breathe into my resistance. I trust there is a deeper place. Instead of rejecting myself, I receive myself and all I am carrying. I let myself feel my discomfort and my yearning at the same time, and I remember that I am capable of making mistakes and growing simultaneously. The more I am able to hold all parts of myself, the more courageous I become in the spiritual assignment of remembering and reclaiming myself beyond whiteness and showing up for the work of love and justice.

- What is your first memory of race?
- What messages did you receive about what it meant to be your race?
- What beliefs and behaviors have you internalized from the culture of white supremacy?
- What has whiteness cost you?
- What are you willing to risk to dismantle white supremacy?
- What practices can you or do you employ to be accountable to yourself and to the broader community?
- What does wellness look like beyond whiteness?

Living into Abolition and Accountability

9/11 was a dividing line in my life. There was everything that came before that moment and everything that came after. But waking up to whiteness was similarly profound. There was who I was when I chose to look the other way—a deeply insecure white woman invested in climbing the ladder and reaping the benefits of my unearned racial privilege. And then there was who I became when I faced the truth and reckoned with my role in white supremacy. Any system that builds you up by tearing other people down will spiritually cost you so much more than what you materially gain. White supremacy robbed me of my relationship to myself and everyone around me. When I came to know myself beyond the delusion of white supremacy, I felt like I belonged—not to some race, but to a community that values all life and believes that our well-being is bound. True well-being was betraying whiteness and reclaiming our collective humanity. So I chose to be a race traitor—to reject the lie of supremacy and the illusion of security and embrace the truth of our mutuality. It means unhooking myself from the attachments of comfort and privilege and turning toward communal connection and care. And it means living a culture of accountability that affirms all life and enables our growth toward a future of collective liberation and well-being.

Accountability only feels like an attack when you're unwilling or unready to acknowledge how your behavior harms others. White supremacy encourages us to protect our own interests, insist on being right, defend our egos, and maintain our sense of importance. Shame keeps us defended and distant, unable to move toward one another, and clinging to good intentions as evidence of our innocence. But intentions do not equal impact. And whether we like it or not, we humans impact each other. Being called out or calling people out is not pleasant. It's often gut wrenching and brutal to the ego. But it is also beautiful in how it affirms that we matter in community. I've come to see callouts as a gift that someone gives me with their time and energy and feedback, and I am learning to receive it with gratitude and action. Accountability is the practice of taking responsibility for the impact of our words and actions, despite our intentions. And while it does not need to be scary, it will be uncomfortable. And it should be.

It's why allyship doesn't go far enough. Allyship is comfortably situated inside a system that is designed for destruction and dehumanization. It is not enough to want to make exploitive, extractive, and violent systems more inclusive. We should want to make them obsolete. True accountability by its very nature should push us outside of our comfort zone—to grow, change, and transform. According to Mia Mingus, there are four key parts to accountability: apologizing, understanding the impact of your actions on yourself and others, making amends, and changing your behavior. That last part is the most important. "True accountability," she says, "is changing your behavior so that the harm, violence, abuse does not happen again."[47]

Which is why we need accountability and justice that goes all the way. Transformative justice seeks to respond to violence without creating more violence and to engage in harm reduction to lessen the violence.* It not only seeks to restore the relationship to its pre-harm state but also to transform the conditions/social structure that created the violence in the first place. Leah Lakshmi Piepzna-Samarasinha describes it as "any way of creating safety, justice and healing for survivors of violence that does not rely on the state" (i.e., prison-industrial complex, criminal legal system, detention centers, foster care, psych hospitals, nursing homes, etc.).[48] Calls for incremental reform are insufficient to address the culture of violence and policing we have inherited, and they have been proven, time and time again, to be ineffective in saving lives and making communities safer. In order to be truly free, we need to disarm the violence that has been normalized in our culture. And that begins with ourselves: What violence and control have we sanctioned? How are we policing each other? Why are we addicted to shaming, blaming, and punishing each other?†

We don't need more cops and cages; we need systems of care and community building. People are safe when they have what they need, when they are not desperate, when they have spaces to heal. Abolition works to build other ways of responding to harms in our society—imagine structures of community care and transformative-justice response teams committed to reparations and reconciliation.‡ It takes its name from the original abolitionists who believed that slavery could not be reformed and must be abolished. When we understand that no one is disposable, then we

---

* Learn more about transformative justice principles in *Beyond Survival*, *Fumbling towards Repair*, and *Love with Accountability*, and follow those who are leading the movement, including Mia Mingus, Leah Lakshmi Piepzna-Samarasinha, Shira Hassan, Ejeris Dixon, Mariame Kaba, and adrienne maree brown.

† Barnard Center for Research on Women created a powerful series of talks called "Building Accountable Communities" featuring the wisdom and experience of transformative and restorative justice practitioners.

‡ An essential abolition reading list: *Abolition for the People* edited by Colin Kaepernick, *We Do This 'til We Free Us* by Mariame Kaba, *Becoming Abolitionists* by Derecka Purnell, and *Abolishing the Police (An Illustrated Introduction)* by Koshka Duff and Cat Sims.

can shift our focus from control and dominance (through policing, prisons, shaming, etc.) to resourcing and repair (through ensuring a living wage, universal healthcare, reparations, etc.). Abolition challenges us to examine how we've been weaponized by white supremacy to police ourselves and one another, so that we can begin decarcerating our minds, bodies, and relationships. And it invites us to practice what we are moving toward: a culture of accountability that is life affirming and whole.

Ruth Wilson Gilmore, professor and prison abolitionist, says, "Abolition is not *absence*, it is *presence*. What the world will become already exists in fragments and pieces, experiments and possibilities.... Abolition is building the future from the present, in all of the ways we can."[49] Abolition is not just about taking action against punitive systems of control such as prisons and immigrant detentions centers (although doing so is vital). It is also about examining the ways we have internalized punitive behaviors in our own lives. We must become abolitionists and dreamers within ourselves and divest from any and all of the ideologies of supremacy and violence that we believe about ourselves and one another. When we uncouple justice from retribution, we can return justice to love and build a country that takes care of everyone.

COLLECTIVE PRACTICE: PRACTICE EVERYDAY ABOLITION

According to Sara Lamble, an organizer with Abolitionist Futures, everyday abolition "is a means to connect efforts toward structural change with our everyday cultures and practices. Everyday abolition means undoing the cultural norms and mindsets that trap us within punitive habits and logics."[50] It calls us to transform the ways we interact with others and to actively change harmful patterns in our daily lives (our homes, our workplaces, our neighborhoods) as well as the systems we are a part of. The following framework from Sarah Lamble and Abolitionist Futures provides four key strategies for everyday abolition:

1. **"Undo carceral cultures: Identify and challenge punitive logics in everyday contexts."** The term *carceral* refers to the logic and practices that equate justice with punishment. These narratives are deeply internalized and require daily work to notice and unhook from them. We can learn to challenge and disrupt such patterns in the moment by developing practices of self-reflection and awareness, not replicating harmful language or behaviors, and building relationships and systems that support consciousness and culture shift.

2. **"Shift from responding to harm with punishment and isolation to offering support, safety, healing, and connection—even when it's hard."** When harm happens, we often respond in one of two ways: by denying or minimizing that harm (this often happens with people we love or to avoid conflict) or by blaming, demonizing, or retaliating. But neither one addresses the root cause of harm or ensures that it doesn't happen again in the future. Instead we need to explore structures of care that respond to harm by practicing love with accountability.[51] This means finding ways to support each other when we or others have done harmful things. It also invites us to look beyond the individual at the broader context and conditions that are contributing to the problem.

3. **"Build our collective skills and capacity to prevent harm and to foster everyday accountability and reparation."** When we build a capacity to identify the early signs of abusive relationships, we learn how to respond to harm without defaulting to defensiveness, punishment, and retaliation. Often one's immediate community (family, friends, neighbors) is much better at intervening in and responding to everyday harm than police or prisons. This means all of us developing new skills around trauma-informed care, safe bystander interventions, conflict resolution, and violence de-escalation.

4. **"Connect everyday practice to broader long-term change."** We need to bridge our everyday practice with social and systemic change to ensure that a world without police and prisons is possible. That means transforming the institutions and structures that normalize punitive culture and policies by supporting campaigns to defund the police, stop prison expansion, challenge the criminal justice system, and redirect funding to community-led efforts that support collective care. It also looks like organizing for housing, healthcare, and racial and economic justice that create the conditions for communities to thrive.

CHAPTER 7

The Politics of Belonging

> Dominator culture has tried to keep us all afraid, to make us choose safety instead of risk, sameness instead of diversity. Moving through that fear, finding out what connects us, revelling in our differences; this is the process that brings us closer, that gives us a world of shared values, of meaningful community.
>
> bell hooks

It's January 29, 2017, and I'm sitting in a room with about 100 other exhausted and scared movement activists. Two days ago, a mere week after his inauguration, Donald Trump issued an executive order banning travel from six Muslim-majority countries to "protect the nation from foreign terrorist entry." While some of us (mainly white people) are shocked by the extreme turn of events, many saw this coming—a culmination of a history of oppression that is yet to be reckoned with. An organizer is speaking about the horrific impact on Muslim and Arab communities, a plight that she says points back to 9/11. My stomach clenches. She describes in detail the post-9/11 discriminatory backlash, the rise in anti-Muslim hate crimes, and the de-Americanization of citizens who were met with suspicion, resentment, and violence. All in the name of 9/11. I felt the hairs on the back of my neck stand up. I became enraged as I realized how people were targeted, harassed, and even killed in Joe's name. After he gave his life for this country, he was used—all of us were used—to justify a war on Arab and Muslim people and crimes against humanity to "make America great again."

I had thought 9/11 was the worst of it—the most unimaginable and devastating loss—but it was just the beginning for so many. Since then, people of Arab and South Asian descent have been intimidated, surveilled, incarcerated, and even killed in exponentially increasing numbers. Many of us were coerced into suspecting our neighbor, buying into stereotypes of who's dangerous and complying with a culture of retaliation. And, as if losing almost 3,000 civilians on 9/11 wasn't enough, it is estimated that nearly 1 million people around the world have been killed due to the "war on terror."[1] Some might say this is the cost of our freedom, but I wondered if it is the price of our fear.

The constant media barrage of images of the towers collapsing was a horror I could not unsee. It was like hypnosis, a constant reminder of what had happened to me and others like me, of how we were wronged. I was expected to be the grieving daughter, the heartbroken New Yorker, the angry American, and I fell in line. The overwhelming praise and homage for the fire department and civil service workers who gave their lives created a sort of fandom and in some strange way implied that my loss, my pain, was more important than what others were going through. That my grief and those who were lost on 9/11 were more worthy and valuable than the lives that were targeted and taken *because of* 9/11. But that story simply fueled our fears and pitted "us" against "them." We played our part and the US got its patriotic war.

The Crisis of Citizenship

Politics has become a dirty word—a forbidden practice that feels too far removed, too corrupt, too unchangeable to the general public. And it's no wonder; one could say that the spirit of American politics has been "trumped" by fanatical politicians and corrupt policies. These days, we leave politics to the pundits, we entrust our well-being to unaccountable politicians, and we stand by while private sector technocrats like Jeff Bezos and Bill Gates meddle in policy. Not only has politics fallen out of alignment with our values and principles, it has fallen out with the people. A recent Princeton University study discovered that if there is zero percent public support for a law, it has a 30 percent likelihood of being passed in Congress. If there is 100 percent public support for a law, it, too, has a 30 percent likelihood of being passed in Congress. In other words, the political preferences of the average American appear to have a "miniscule, statistically non-significant impact on public policy."[2] That's why things like background checks for gun owners (84 percent public support), Medicare for all (70 percent public support), higher taxes for the rich (64 percent public support), and reducing pollution (80 percent public support) have all but stalled in Congress.[3]

But it's no wonder. American democracy has been crowded out by bureaucracy and corruption. Take money in politics, which, without campaign finance reform, leaves candidates vulnerable to billionaires and corporate lobbying. Or a two-party system, which makes it impossible for other parties to compete (even while almost 50 percent identify as independent).[4] Or gerrymandering, which gives politicians the ability to rig their districts in their favor. Or voter suppression, which deliberately discourages and disenfranchises voters. All of this adds up to a failed political system that is no longer considered a full democracy by political think tanks and analysts like the Economic Intelligence Unit. Is the system broken? Yes. But while it is easy to point the finger at institutional power for our failing democracy, we rarely talk about the other, also broken component of our political system—citizenship.

The US language of democracy has always included the essential role of citizens.* It declared that our rights were natural and inalienable, but it was intended that the American people animate and defend that declaration.

---

* Eric Liu has written some great books on reimagining citizenship including *The Gardens of Democracy, Become America,* and *You Are More Powerful Than You Think.*

There was responsibility implied in our founding documents, a social pact so to speak. But after more than 200 years of impassioned civic duty—the kind that people fought for, the kind that people died for—things have changed. Since the 1970s, all indicators of civic life, from volunteering to neighborliness to social connectedness, have declined.[5] More and more of us are becoming more siloed in our bubbles, distracted by our devices, and dislodged from our place in society. In other words, people have stopped engaging with one another in community. Instead, we transact in siloed spaces (yoga studios, health food co-ops, meditation groups), which only reinforces self interest and us-vs.-them behavior.

And the hyperindividualized wellness craze isn't helping. We opt for personalized wellness regimens over public health options. We build net-zero houses but don't insist on environmental protection laws. We value farm-to-table foods but don't advocate for the farmers who actually harvest the food. When Carol Hanisch said "the personal is political" in 1969, she wasn't talking about organic shampoo. She was responding to the isolation that women experienced around gender oppression. "There are no personal solutions at this time. There is only collective action for a collective solution."[6] In other words, our problems are not personal so much as they are structural, which means they demand a structural response. But these days, the phrase is used to imply the opposite: that taking uncoordinated individual actions—like composting, taking shorter showers, changing out light bulbs, buying organic, "voting with your dollar"—somehow constitutes political action.* Not only does this not achieve structural transformation, but it reinforces the toxic independence and individualism that are undermining our collective survival.

The concept of citizenship, when invoked these days, is reduced to xenophobic debates about immigration restrictions instead of our shared responsibility to democracy. And we have a right to feel discouraged; money in politics has enabled a marketplace of democracy that allows votes to be bought and sold to the highest bidder. But not only are voters treated like

---

* In *Hegemony How To: A Roadmap for Radicals* Jonathan Smucker provides a practical guide for how to build community power through culture shift and grassroots organizing.

consumers, we often act like it. Our "what's in it for me" mentality conspires to keep us feeling powerless. When we see ourselves as consumers, we engage through the lens of cynicism, suspicion, and selfishness. We begin to believe that our needs can be best determined and met by the actions of others, whether that is corporations, elected officials, social service providers, and so forth. Wellness culture feeds that ideology by convincing us that we can't be well or empowered unless we subscribe to the latest self-help prescription or submit to the hot new clean diet. It invites us to sit comfortably on our meditation cushions, mastering calm while waiting around for someone else to solve our problems.

The echoes of America's founding wounds—colonization, individualism, white supremacy—leave us fending for ourselves, protecting our power and position, and abandoning our neighbors. It looks like a citizenship from the sidelines—a culture of finger-pointing, fair-weather voting, and expecting someone else to take care of things. But no one is coming to save us. Our collective well-being is only possible with the realization of all its parts.

Who Belongs Here?

The United States was founded by immigrants who, without claim or documentation, literally declared themselves naturalized in 1776. My eleventh great-grandfather Edward Ketcham was a founding settler. He came over as an indentured servant in 1629, trading his freedom for transport to North America. Unlike many ancestors of color, my white ancestors would not only get free but end up accumulating considerable wealth and status throughout their life, an inheritance that I benefit from to this day. But not all of our ancestors came here of their own free will. Indigenous ancestors were here before Europeans invaded this continent, many African ancestors were abducted and brought to America by force, and some Mexican ancestors experienced the border crossing *them* when lines were redrawn following the Mexican-American War. No matter how we got here, who gets to belong and who doesn't has been a question we've been asking in America all along.

Racism and misogyny were codified into America's very first immigration law. The Naturalization Act of 1790 reserved naturalized citizenship for "free white person[s] . . . of good character."[7] This excluded most women, Native Americans, indentured servants, and enslaved and free Africans. Black Americans were not granted US citizenship until 1868, which would turn out to be conditional at best given Jim Crow. Women weren't granted full citizenship independent of their husbands until 1922. And Native Americans weren't considered citizens until 1924, despite living here for millennia. Throughout our history, the laws and ideas about citizenship have shape-shifted to privilege and protect those deemed "fit" for the American project and worthy of belonging. That debate over who gets to be American lives on today.

These days, to be without citizenship is not only to be without basic rights and protections but to live with the fear of family separation and deportation. The 11 million undocumented people in the US aren't just immigrants, they are essential. Nearly three in four undocumented immigrants work on the front lines to keep the country moving forward. They pay taxes often without receiving the protections and benefits that tax dollars afford to citizens, such as welfare, food stamps, Medicaid, and emergency relief (e.g., they were excluded from all federal COVID relief plans).[8] Despite playing an essential role in the American economy and way of life, undocumented immigrants face substantial economic and legal barriers to accessing healthcare, are ineligible for public insurance, and are excluded from basic safety-net support. But Jose Antonio Vargas, undocumented activist and author of *Dear America: Notes of an Undocumented Citizen*, points out, "We are here because you were there," referencing how decades of US imperialism created the conditions where people need to flee and seek a better life elsewhere.[9] The US's history of intervention has cut deep wounds in neighboring countries, making it harder for people to survive; upon arrival they meet America's brutal border policies, ongoing surveillance, incarceration, and worse.*

---

* *Dear America: Notes of an Undocumented Citizen* by Jose Antonio Vargas is a powerful memoir about being undocumented and othered and the true meaning of citizenship.

But our borders haven't always been closed. Ellis Island was an open border through which 12 million people passed, two of whom were my ancestors Emelio and Carmella Raffio, who migrated from southern Italy in 1910. All that was required for entry was the name of the ship they came on, their intention for staying, and a medical examination (to ensure they would be healthy, able, and productive). They arrived just in time, before the Immigration Act of 1924 restricted immigration from Southern and Eastern Europe and specifically sought to exclude Jewish people (who were referred to at the time as the lowest of all European races).[10] When signing the legislation into law, President Calvin Coolidge declared that "America must be kept American."[11]

Nearly 100 years later, that call echoed through the nation once again under a campaign that promised to deport Mexican immigrants, ban Muslims and others who come from "shithole" countries, and build a wall.[12] But "Make America Great Again" simply means "Make America White Again," the definition of which would be adapted throughout history to accommodate white power. Immigrants like my Irish and Italian ancestors, who were willing and able to attain whiteness, were not only afforded the benefits of citizenship (like voting rights, jobs, and education) but were granted belonging, status, and protection. Membership to this top rung of the racial caste ladder would forever be used to divide us and pit us against each other. It is the central conflict of this country—are we an America where all people belong? Or are we an America that belongs only to white, straight, wealthy, nondisabled men?

Divide-and-Conquer Politics

November 9, 2016, was like waking up to a nightmare. Like many, I was not surprised that Trump had won. I had been canvassing for weeks and witnessed firsthand that many were falling for Trump's scare tactics and fear mongering. What I wasn't prepared for that next day was the fear and despair around what was to come in Trump's America. Never before had I felt targeted by a system that intended to harm me and the people I love. It exposed my comfort and privilege in a whole new way. But Trump wasn't the beginning of xenophobia and fascism, nor would he be the end. And many of us would painfully discover that Trump was not different from us; he was simply the worst of us, embodying our greed for more, our fear of the "other," our narcissism and obsession with ourselves, and our disconnection from ourselves and one another. What transpired over the next four years was not just a reckoning with a wannabe dictator, it was a reckoning with ourselves. Election Day 2016 was the day America woke up to the wound that had been festering for more than 400 years. Trump's election was not a new diagnosis. It was the wound reopened, the flesh exposed, the rank unleashed. And a big part of the heartbreak and fear that many of us felt was the knowledge, somewhere deep down, that we were complicit, that we had let it happen.

America was built on the ground of divide and conquer. The history of dispossession, enslavement, and white supremacy was not inevitable but strategic and purposeful in the pursuit of freedom and wealth for white people. This push and pull has been at the heart of US politics since the beginning. It traces back to 1675, when Nathaniel Bacon united commoners (both English and African) in a rebellion against the exploits of the elite class and the advances of Indigenous Peoples. Though unsuccessful, this cross-racial alliance posed a threat that shook the governing class to such an extent that they created a new social status based on race that would privilege white workers and relegate people of African descent to a lifetime (and inheritance) of slavery.[13] From there, every step in the direction of racial justice and liberation would be met with resistance. The abolition of slavery was met with a wave of racialized terror in the form of lynchings across the former slave states. After reconstruction, Jim Crow swept in to subjugate and disenfranchise free Black men for almost 100 years. Following the great strides of the civil rights movement of the 1960s, the government responded with a call for "law and order" that targeted Black Americans and resulted in the largest system of incarceration in the world. And after eight years of being led by the first Black president in US history, America elected a wannabe fascist dictator in an effort to "make America great again."

Divide and conquer continues to be the wedge that prevents a cross-racial working class movement toward justice and collective well-being. It weaponizes racism to effectively separate people whose shared interests remain a significant threat to elite power. It seduces white people with false promises of personal freedom and security in the face of demoralizing poverty and the denial of essential social services reserved for the rich and powerful. In this system, poor white people don't own the table, but they're coerced to uphold it, to guard the gate of social and institutional power with the false hope that it will protect them. Their cause is fueled by a manufactured fear—fear of losing out to the so-called other. This cocktail, made worse by economic insecurity, environmental instability, and racial entitlement, creates a perfect storm that leaves many vulnerable to disinformation and divide-and-conquer tactics that pit us against each other instead of uniting us in collective survival. Keeping people in a perpetual state of scarcity, convincing them that resources are denied to them because of [insert scapegoat racial group], only serves to distract people from the real source of their suffering: systems of power and wealth accumulation.*

This us-vs.-them strategy asserts that "they" are a threat to "us." "They" are dangerous and must be controlled, contained, or converted. "They" are bringing drugs, "they" are committing crimes, "they" are stealing our jobs, "they" are terrorists, "they" are a drain on society. When people buy into the concept of supremacy, equal rights for everyone can feel like an attack on some people's freedom. But it was never freedom for everyone but rather freedom for a subset of people in power that has taken precedence over all other things—even other people's safety, dignity, and well-being. According to this story, this country has only ever belonged to some people (white, Christian, English-speaking, etc.) and everyone else is a threat to that cause. Heather McGhee, author of *The Sum of Us*, writes, "The zero-sum paradigm lingers as more than a story justifying an economic order; it also animates many people's sense of who is an American,

---

* One of my favorite books on why we're divided and what it's costing us is *Sum of Us: What Racism Costs Everyone and How We Can Prosper Together* by Heather McGhee, who proves that racism is working against all of us.

and whether more rights for other people will come at the expense of their own."[14]

I feel the toxicity of this logic in my own body. It is the stories I grew up with that told me to strive and compete and fight for my place in the world. It is the belief that I am never enough and there is not enough to go around. It is the fear of losing ground that encourages me to cling to and protect what I have. It is how I learned to distrust the other, as if someone else's thriving and success were at the expense of my own. It is the lie of whiteness that afforded me countless privileges at the expense of others. It is the false promise of well-being as something that is separate from the people and planet around me. It is all of the constructed myths that have pitted us against each other and prevented us from working together to build systems that take care of everyone. And now, faced with the impending doom of an ecological crisis and an uncertain future, it is stirring a shared chronic anxiety that is making many of us susceptible to inadequate solutions to increasingly complex problems, where divide and distract, blame and shame, us vs. them becomes the dominant method for how we cope.

Politicians have long preyed upon people's anxiety and fear about marginalized people to win elections and advance their political agendas. Racial narratives are created and exploited by people in power to deflect responsibility for social and economic insecurity to the "other" and hijack the government for their own benefit. Everything is about race and power but is coded as if it's not. In *Dog Whistle Politics: How Coded Appeals Have Reinvented Racism and Wrecked the Middle Class*, Ian Haney López, professor of law at the University of California, Berkeley, exposes the coded racial appeals that are weaponized by politicians to instill fear and sow division. A "dog whistle" means speaking in code to a target audience, such as using phrases like "forced busing," "welfare queen," "inner city crime," and "illegal immigrant" in ways that carry racist subtexts.[15] And as a future where white people no longer occupy the majority approaches (by 2045), this sort of rhetoric is getting louder, more manipulative, and more vicious by the day—and it laid the groundwork for a tyrant to come in, stoke the fears of millions of people, and promise to lock up, deport, and punish the bogeyman.[16] Trump was the personification of divisiveness: a lying, insulting, press-bashing, racist demagogue who boasted of grabbing pussy, praised dictators and nationalists, and sabotaged American democracy. Anat Shenker-Osorio, messaging expert and host of the podcast *Words to Win By*, elaborates on the cost of invoking fear: "Dog whistling is not merely about creating ill will towards communities of color. It's about cementing the notion that we cannot have an 'us,' we cannot have a collective, we cannot have shared things. We cannot have a universal single-payer health care system; we cannot have paid time to care for our families; we cannot have labor protection that cover us all—we can't have an us because there's a them.... Dog whistle politics at its core is about undermining the collective."[17]

At the core of our predicament is an ideology of separation, scarcity, and supremacy that plays on our fears and manipulates us into blaming people below us in the hierarchy of bodies for our struggles. According to Umair Haque, "The people who expected and felt entitled to lives of safety, security and stability—who anticipated being at the top of a tidy little hierarchy, the boss of this or that, the chieftain of that or this, but now find themselves adrift and unmoored in a collapsing society, powerless . . . they turn to those who promise them just that superiority by turning on those below them."[18] Unemployed? That's because immigrants are taking your jobs. Addicted? That's because Black people are selling drugs. Which only distracts people from recognizing the real problem: the increasing concentration of wealth and power by an elite few. Because if we were to acknowledge the imbalance of power that is breeding inequality and denying so many the resources and conditions needed to thrive, we could unite in collective solidarity to challenge the status quo.

In a better world, perhaps, we would celebrate the increasing diversity of our American family. In this world, however, we are likely to devolve further into division and the delusion of white replacement theory. In the face of a perceived "racial threat," many white people build walls and forbid history related to racism from being taught in the classroom. Some (in the wellness world especially) fall prey to conspiracy theories that liken mask mandates and social safety policies to "crimes against humanity." Others rewrite the rules of democracy to protect the dominant group through voter suppression laws, gerrymandering, and outright insurrection.[19] Fueled by the rhetoric of xenophobia (and amplified by social media), modern fascism has quickly expanded to prey on the panic and fear of white America. But while dominant culture may be trying to divide us, well-being is calling us back together. Not through sameness, but through the "sum of us."

Why We Need Identity Politics

Inevitably, in moments of division and fear—like after 9/11 or the 2021 Capitol insurrection—there are calls for "unity" by way of ignoring difference and bypassing harm. "It's past time for all of us to try and heal our country and move forward," said Senator Lindsey Graham after the attacks on the Capitol.[20] While conflict makes us uncomfortable, unity is seductive. It invites us to rise above the complex mess that is our national identity and find "common ground." But calls for unity without truth and accountability only uphold the status quo. Yvette Simpson put it best when she said: "Unity is great, but freedom is better. And there is the part of this population that has sacrificed their freedom time and time again.... I want the kind of unity that leads to change for the people who have waited for it."[21]

Calls for civility politics—using language like "unity," "common ground," and "we're all in it together"—invite us to glaze over difference and bypass the discomfort that accompanies it. But naming differences isn't what creates division. Despite our shared humanity, we are each having a very different experience of being alive on the planet right now. Each person's safety, belonging, and dignity are determined by a hierarchy of bodies that is designed for the well-being of some at the expense of others. In most spaces, conflict emerges when recognizing these truths becomes too much to handle. This is especially true in wellness culture, where leaders often insist on "safe spaces" that silence conflict and promise positive vibes only. But ignoring difference and the very real lived experiences of those who are marginalized only protects the comfort of those who are already safe. There can be no neutral, no safety, no "manifest your reality" in a system designed to keep only some people well. Everything is political, especially our well-being.

Author and cofounder of Black Lives Matter Alicia Garza points out that "the reason that people don't want to talk about identity, is because they want to obscure how power is actually functioning and operating. And this notion that to talk about race or to talk about gender is divisive, is really to say, 'I don't want you to expose unequal distribution of power that I've received at your expense.'"[22] All of the most divisive issues in recent history—police shootings of unarmed Black men, religious exemptions from discrimination law, the right of trans people to "exist in public" (in the words of Laverne Cox[23]), sexual harassment, and rape culture—have all been described as "identity politics." These are all issues in which communities that have been targeted by oppression are speaking truth to power and exposing inequality.

The term *identity politics* was coined by the Combahee River Collective in 1974. In what would become one of the most important Black feminist texts, they argued that "the most profound and potentially most radical politics come directly out of our own identity, as opposed to working to end somebody else's oppression."[24] The concept emerged to confront the politics of sameness being perpetuated by second wave feminism that assumed that all women's experiences were the same. They're not. This bold statement laid the groundwork for intersectional feminism, which understands that all systems of oppression are interlocking.* The concept was developed further by critical race theory scholar Kimberlé Crenshaw, who describes intersectionality as "a prism for seeing the way in which various forms of inequality often operate together and exacerbate each other."[25] It's not just a lens through which we understand how we're shaped by our intersecting identities; it is a call to follow the lead of those most affected by injustice and trust the solutions that emerge from their lived experience and wisdom.

Of course, the identity you hear the least about is white (and cis, male, straight, wealthy, and nondisabled) identity. As Garza puts it, "Identity is

---

* Keeanga-Yamahtta Taylor curates interviews and essays with the founding members of the Combahee River Collective and contemporary activists to reflect on the legacy of the statement and its impact on Black feminism and today's struggles in *How We Get Free: Black Feminism and the Combahee River Collective*.

only important when—through no fault of your own—you are assigned an identity that promises worse life outcomes" than those in power.[26] Rarely do people in power take issue with the fact that a different— dominant—identity politics is in fact shaping all of our lives. And most of us are suffering because of it. Issues pertaining to white identity get normalized as everyone's issues—the standard by which all progress is measured. And when our politics is organized around what white people need, how white people are suffering, and what white people value, too many are left behind. All of this sets us up for a zero-sum game of winners and losers and not being the one to get left behind. Which is exactly what identity politics is asking: For whom is progress being made? Who is most likely to live in poverty? Who is most likely to die in childbirth? Who is most likely to be unemployed? Who is most likely to be shot by police? Who is most likely to be denied the right to vote? The privilege to not see or acknowledge these disparities contributes to the delusion and divisiveness that is holding us back.*

The truth behind these questions is why identity politics is needed. Critiques of identity politics only arise when people in power feel threatened by a focus on identities that are not their own. They claim that the culture of political correctness, callouts, and cancellations is dividing us. But the real "cancel culture" is that of abject poverty and mass incarceration and workplace discrimination, where entire groups of people are systemically stifled and silenced from participation. Movements like #MeToo and #BlackLivesMatter simply expose systems that protect the elite at the expense of entire peoples, and they have effectively used social media to hold people accountable. These online reckonings reflect the voice of a people who are breaking their silence to stop the cycle of harm—and in the absence of systems of accountability, they are needed.†

---

* Alicia Garza explores identity politics and how to build transformative movement power in *The Purpose of Power: How We Come Together When We Fall Apart.*

† In *We Will Not Cancel Us: And Other Dreams of Transformative Justice*, adrienne maree brown grapples with cancel culture and offers abolition dreams that point us in the direction of alternative ways to navigate harm and accountability.

We don't know how to hold conflict in our culture. Instead, we default to us-vs.-them strategies that diminish people's identities and lived experiences. Identity politics seeks to correct that by exposing how identity has been constructed and maintained throughout history to determine who gets to be well, and how identity-based oppression and harm have accumulated and compounded over generations to hold entire groups of people back. Identity politics gives us a way to disrupt a dominant narrative that denies the whole of who we are and prevents us from tapping into our full human potential. Identity politics is a bridge, not a divide.

Apathy Kills

In the weeks after the 2016 election, I was invited to a number of house parties as folks struggled to navigate that moment. People were reckoning with questions like "How could this have happened?" and "What more could I have done?" and were looking to community leaders and organizers who could shed light on how we got here and where we go next. The most common thing I heard in living rooms and at kitchen tables was people's obsession with the family member who voted for Trump. Our conversation was dominated by the desire for tactics to help them go get their uncle or cousin. After a few of these experiences, I tried an experiment. I asked them to make a list of everyone they knew who had voted for Trump. For many it was two to six people. Then I asked them to make a list of everyone they knew who had, since the election, gone back to "normal." That list was more like twenty-five to forty. And that's when I understood what we were up against. It wasn't a war against political extremism. It was a war against political apathy.

Apathy works like a chemical reaction. It's not so much that people simply do not care and, therefore, do not engage. Rather it is an embodied trauma response that occurs when we are unable to tolerate the feelings associated with a situation. Apathy is a learned disconnection, fostered through the numbing of Netflix or the distraction of fake news or the busying of our busy lives. We become seduced by distraction to avoid discomfort. It is one of the body's primal defense moves when it senses a real or perceived threat to its safety. Of course, our sense of safety is precarious at best these days. In the face of growing economic insecurity, environmental threats, racial violence, fascist leadership, and an uncertain future, it makes sense that many of us are susceptible to numbing out and shutting down to cope with our chronic anxiety.

But when apathy intersects with powerlessness, fear of conflict, and self-righteousness, it turns toxic. How else did we get to a place where so many are disengaged and distracted? Where we see undeniable evidence of climate change and do nothing to alter our footprint. Where we can allow hundreds of thousands to die needlessly from a pandemic and not demand accountability. Where we can scroll past the news of another unjust police killing, or another mass shooting, or another murdered trans woman of color, and not feel the heartbreak viscerally. While the overwhelming nature of our predicament is understandable, it's not an excuse. Apathy kills.

So much time is spent debating civility politics and how to reach across the aisle to work together, but these debates miss the point entirely. The real divide isn't between the right and left. The real divide is between political junkies and everyone else. A recent poll found that upward of 80 to 85 percent of people follow politics casually or not at all.[27] In other words, most of us are too busy or too overwhelmed or too self-interested to engage in democracy. I spent most of my life politically disengaged and uninterested in the well-being of people outside of my bubble. Wellness culture promised that if I focused on transforming myself and my personal footprint, the world would be a better place. It sells electric cars, net-zero homes, and organic beauty products as the answer to systemic and catastrophic crises. It suggests autoimmune boosters and plant-based diets in response to a pandemic. But assuaging our fears through alternative solutions and personal antidotes reinforces our distrust in systems of government and each other. And that is the very thing that triggers apathy.

Fear of conflict is deeply embedded in dominant culture, causing us to avoid uncomfortable conversations, deflect confrontation, and give in to toxic positivity. While intolerance for conflict is often masked as "respect-ability politics," its impact only reinforces the status quo. Our unwillingness to engage in conflict stems from an attachment to ego, status, control, and power. It is evident in how so many of us call 911 to resolve conflict with our neighbors, depend on law enforcement and incarceration to hold people accountable, and defer to politicians and elected officials to make the rules for society. Fear of conflict is also related to how so many of us distance ourselves from community and connection, numb and shield ourselves from the impact of being humans in relationship, and wall ourselves off in gated communities. It is this defended state that enables us to become bystanders in the face of injustice. But bystanders are not neutral. Our unwillingness to disrupt, speak out, and confront is what allows patterns of abuse to continue.

Elie Wiesel said that "the opposite of love is not hate, it's indifference."[28] Apathy is acceptance of the unacceptable, resigning ourselves to "that's just how things are." But it's not just a mindset, it's a trauma response in the face of overwhelming issues, where individuals lose the capacity to feel and act. But what about when apathy afflicts an entire population? Many of us seem to have strong political opinions in private and rarely act on them in public. Social media has given us the power to exercise our activism from the comfort of our computers and phones, but it can also make us less likely to engage beyond the screen—less likely to join protests, lobby for change, vote in local elections, and hold political leaders accountable. Simply holding political views or reacting to political events is not the same thing as being political. Political action demands interventions that redistribute power, transform structures, and reshape the world. Everything else is just commentary.

All of this adds up to a citizenship of privilege and neglect that is making Americans unwell—and is going to make our species extinct. It is the supremacy of entitlement, the scarcity of hoarding, and the separation from our mutuality that allow the rich to keep getting richer, the preservation of private healthcare and schools (at the expense of public options), and the continued extraction of natural resources (causing catastrophic climate change). There is no political path forward without moving through the deep wounds of separation, scarcity, and supremacy that have shaped us collectively and held us back from living up to our potential. True citizenship invites us to come together in both shared struggle and shared goals, so that we can work toward a politics of collective well-being. The government is us. It is our dysfunctional family gone sideways at Thanksgiving, and we must reclaim our role as citizens and cocreate an American Dream that has never been. That means not just confronting the conflict and division but creating the conditions for belonging and participation that enable everyone to thrive. We need a citizenship of solidarity—one that centers love, interdependence, and the idea that no one is well unless everyone is well. It's not solidarity for the sake of the other. It's solidarity for the sake of all of us.

RECOVERY

People are aware that they cannot continue in the same old way but are immobilized because they cannot imagine an alternative. We need a vision that recognizes that we are at one of the great turning points in human history when the survival of our planet and the restoration of our humanity require a great sea change in our ecological, economic, political, and spiritual values.

GRACE LEE BOGGS

It's September 15, 2016, and I'm standing at a gas station in Mesa, Arizona. I was brought here by my friend Valarie Kaur, an activist and filmmaker, whose story collided with mine months earlier. It is an unlikely site for a memorial, transformed by white sheets that are draped over the asphalt and flowers that adorn a marble memorial. A crowd gathers around the memorial while drivers continue to pull in and pump gas. Next to me is Rana Singh Sodhi, who is telling me about the life and death of his brother, Balbir Singh Sodhi. You likely have not heard of him—his name was barely mentioned in the media. He was not mourned by the nation. But he, like my stepdad, was a man beloved by his family and friends, a man of God and of service to his community. And, like Joe, he was another soul unnecessarily taken from us.

Four days after 9/11, while my family was weeding through the rubble, Balbir Sodhi was trying to figure out how he could help out the victims of 9/11. He was a good man, Rana tells me of his older brother. He knew the risk to Sikh and Muslim Americans in the aftermath of 9/11 and told his brother to stay home. But he himself was determined to do something. That morning, as he was planting flowers in front of the gas station where he worked to honor the lives of those lost just days earlier, wearing a beard and a turban in accordance with his Sikh faith, he was shot five times in the back by a white man who claimed to act in the name of patriotism. Balbir was the first American to be killed in a hate crime in the aftermath of 9/11, but he would most certainly not be the last.[29] Countless innocent lives were lost not just on 9/11 but *because of it.*

It made me wonder whether, despite the vows to "never forget" what happened on 9/11, we are really remembering when we don't tell the whole story. The one that includes the suffering of so many who have been unjustly persecuted since that day. And am I truly honoring the memory of the man who raised me, who demonstrated a love for his neighbors every day of his life? Joe wasn't a superhero. He, like Balbir and so many that day, was an ordinary person who did an extraordinary thing. I think that is the legacy they leave us—that we are all ordinary people who can do extraordinary things for each other and for the future that we all belong to.

For years, Valarie and I had told two heartbreaking versions of the same event. Eventually our stories became one, woven together in such a way that they could no longer be separate. Fifteen years after 9/11, we came together at Ground Zero, the place where it all began. This time, we brought with us the story of Balbir Sodhi and the many innocent people that had been taken since 9/11. Four days later, we traveled across the country to the memorial at the gas station that had become known as the second Ground Zero. We brought with us the story of Lt. Joseph Leavey and all the courageous first responders who gave their lives on 9/11. We stood in solidarity, side by side, hand in hand, hearts on the line, two unlikely allies who embodied a revolutionary kind of love that transcended race, religion, and politics. While it was our suffering that united us, it was our relationship that transformed us.*

After fifteen years of trying to honor Joe's memory and live up to the sacrifice he made for all of us, I realized that all that I was seeking for healing and transformation was right there in my relationship with Valarie and Rana. How there is no healing in half-truths, incomplete stories, and broken bonds. And there is no recovery from the wound of 9/11 or any of the wounds of our collective history unless we locate ourselves in the larger

---

* Valarie Kaur writes about her experience as a Sikh American in the aftermath of 9/11 in *See No Stranger: A Memoir and Manifesto of Revolutionary Love.*

story of who we are and show up for the well-being of everyone. Balbir's story taught me that we belong to each other. Our stories, like our healing, are inseparable. And if giving in to fear and division is what got us here, opening to courage and belonging is what will heal us forward.

True well-being calls us to turn toward one another with courage and compassion, so that we can build a world where everyone belongs. It is an everyday practice of showing up for the bigger *we* and the future that we all deserve. And this is where well-being and politics converge. When we organize our lives around collective care, we can work together to build the systems and structures needed for collective safety, belonging, and dignity. Only then can we create a new story of us that rises to the occasion and reimagines a future where we can all be well.

From Us vs. Them to *We*

I come from a long line of first responders. My birth father, like my step-father, comes from many generations of "water carriers," or firefighters who risked their lives for the community. And while my dad and I shared a commitment to public service, we didn't share the same politics. I discovered the rift during the 2012 presidential election. Tensions were high as Republicans were trying desperately to unseat the first Black president. While I came in fired up about Obama's policies, my dad told a different story, one of increasing economic hardship and cultural estrangement. For three days, we dug in, both fully invested in our own story and unwilling to cede territory to the other. I left that trip feeling disappointed and betrayed. How could we be so close and yet so far apart? Despite my silence, my dad called often, leaving messages, always kind and curious. When I finally got up the courage to call years later, my dad asked what happened. I didn't know how to answer. How to tell him that I moved away from him because I couldn't tolerate his beliefs, I couldn't hear his story of fear and belonging, I couldn't see him in his vulnerability. Then my dad said the most profound thing: "I didn't understand why you wouldn't speak to me. Because I see you out there speaking your truth and standing up for what you believe in and I love you more, not less." I learned a lot from him that day—that love is what happens not despite your differences but because of them. While my dad and I didn't find common ground, we did find a way to see each other across our differences and meet each other with empathy and love.

While many of the problems of today are not new, the pace and magnitude of what we are facing—with changing demographics, technology, globalization, and climate—are unprecedented. We can only process so much change in a short period without experiencing significant anxiety and dissonance regarding existential questions about who we are and who we are becoming. Threats, both real and imagined, can trigger irrational responses (flight, fight, freeze) that immobilize and pit us against each other. Without the capacity to work with our fear and move through our discomfort, we become vulnerable to dog-whistle narratives, disinformation campaigns, absurd conspiracy theories, and demagogues.* Our anxieties can lead us to hoard resources, defend our turf, and dream of getting "back to normal." Even striving toward wellness can be a trauma response when we're not paying attention. From compulsive spiritual seeking, relentless self-improvement, and perfectionism, I found myself increasingly disconnected from relationships and from reality itself. But this story—that our well-being is separate from or supreme to others'—is not only a myth but is the very thing that is keeping us stuck.

Stories are powerful. At their best, they imagine new and better worlds that we can aspire to. At their worst, they exploit our pain and vulnerability for profits and power. Regardless of their intention, stories shape our reality. In America we've inherited a legacy of division—a dominant story that was constructed to break us apart, turn us against the land and each other, and justify supremacy and oppression. This story is expressed through every facet of society. It is alive in all of us, shaping our words and actions, training us to play our prescribed role and maintain the status quo. At the core of our complicity is fear for our well-being and an assumption that it is being threatened by the "other." When we "other" one another, we don't just turn

---

* Zach Norris offers a vision for addressing and preventing harm to break the cycles of fear, violence, and trauma by investing in collective care in *Defund Fear: Safety without Policing, Prisons and Punishment.*

against each other, we turn inward. We separate and seek refuge in isolation. We escape the harsh realities of our shared experience by retreating into meditation, getting drawn to conspiracy theories, and insisting on positive vibes only. We hoard resources and demand special treatment and exclusive cures. And we buy into a myth that there can be a "well-being of me" at the expense of the "well-being of we." This myth is at the very heart of our suffering because it demands that we forget the truth of our interdependence: that there is no healing outside of each other—no magic pill or exotic ritual, no juice fast or yoga fad, no meditation or retreat—that can heal the wound that has cut us off from one another and the whole of who we are.

The science of safety supports this theory. Faced with a rapidly changing, ever threatening world, the modern nervous system is on high alert, scanning its environment to answer three fundamental questions: Am I safe? Do I belong? Do they accept me? The vagus nerve (the longest nerve in the body) operates like air traffic control, observing, processing, and responding at all times and determining how to best react to danger and mobilize the rest of the body. But in a state of acceleration such as ours, exacerbated by a culture of fear, the nervous system gets stuck in a chronic state of defense. In other words, how we react to each other much of the time is ruled by our nervous system's fight, flight, or freeze response.[30] But this is where a wellness movement that is committed to collective well-being could really help us—by offering practices that regulate the nervous system, disarm our defenses, and increase our capacity to reach out in compassion and connection.

And it's more than self-regulation, it is co-regulation. The paradox of our human condition is that we are wired for both safety and connection. On a biological level, safety simply means that our bodies are not in a chronic state of high alert—not constantly scanning to see if we are OK, if we belong, and if we are valued. The irony is that this sense of safety doesn't come from self-preservation or individual protection; rather, it's a result of deepening relationships and caring for others—and being cared for in return. Finding safe sources of social engagement in the face of fear not only reorients the body to feel safe, calm, and connected, but it heals the old response patterns and survival shaping, so that we can practice a new way of being together. That's right—reaching out to each other and building relationships recalibrates our nervous system from defense to embrace, from fear to ease, from apathy to empathy.

While apathy calls us to turn inward and away, empathy invites us to turn toward each other. Empathy is seeing ourselves in one another. But it goes beyond connecting with another person's pain. Mark Gonzales, of the Department of the Future, defines empathy as a "worldview that sees everyone as a degree of self." Deep empathy, he says, is embracing the full spectrum of another person's experience, which includes their pain *and* their joy.[31] It is understanding the cause and effect of our interconnected lives. When I heard Valarie's story, I realized that if it were not for the death of my stepfather, the life of Balbir would still exist. Our stories were intrinsically tied, in the same way that one person's privilege can never be separated from another's oppression, nor my well-being uncoupled from yours.

Detoxing from apathy is turning our attention to each other and embracing conflict with curiosity and compassion. It is building the human capacity to show up not despite our differences but because of them, learning how to change together and, ultimately, how to belong to each other. That means asking hard questions about who's missing and what it's gonna take to build a future where everyone belongs. Instead of othering, we can begin "bridging"—identifying the values and needs that are underneath the surface and looking for not just common ground but human ground.[32] It's learning that we can disagree with each other and still love each other. Because making the shift from apathy to empathy, from othering to belonging, has enormous consequences, not just for our present well-being but for our collective survival.

There are few things as central to our human identity and well-being as belonging.* Feelings of belonging influence one's identity and the extent to which one feels accepted, valued, and able to take on a role in society. Belonging is not the same as inclusion, which can exist within

---

* *Redefining Who Belongs* is a publication by the Othering and Belonging Institute that puts forth narrative strategies that disrupt the culture of us vs. them and reimagines a new story of "us": https://belonging.berkeley.edu/redefining-who-belongs.

(and reinforce) power structures and dominant stories. Rather, belonging defies those paradigms and says that we belong simply because we are. Belonging is both inherent and shared. It affirms that each of us has a right to be here and that we are all a necessary part of the whole. Belonging does not create borders or build walls. It does not deny our difference or encourage sameness. It understands that while we may be situated in different locations within dynamic systems of oppression, our destiny is bound.

And yet many of us are scrambling to find a true sense of belonging. When I look back at my own journey, I can see now that I was always simply trying to get home again. From my parents' divorce to climbing the corporate ladder to healing from 9/11 to finding my purpose to becoming an activist, it has all been a desperate attempt to arrive at some mythical destination and feel worthy of belonging. But the belief that belonging was something I had to buy or take or earn was the very thing that kept me from it. Only when I learned that "we can be home for each other," as my friend Teo Drake says— that we belong to each other—was I able to slow down and see that what I had been searching and yearning for was all around me. Home is not a place but a state of belonging. And the practice of citizenship is how we take care of our shared home.

A citizen is "one who is willing to be accountable for and committed to the well-being of the whole," Peter Block says. "Choosing to be accountable for the whole, creating a context of hospitality and collective possibility, acting to bring the gifts of those on the margin into the center—these are some of the ways we begin to create a community of citizens."[33] It isn't about papers or where you come from or what language you speak. It's how you show up and make a contribution to the whole of who we are. Citizenship is something that many of us take for granted. Those of us who were born into the "American ideal" never had to fight for the belonging and privileges associated with citizenship. It wasn't anything we earned, we just were. Over time, we may have adopted a "what's in it for me" attitude rather than "what's my part to play." Those who have been denied the privileges of full citizenship, however, on the grounds of race, class, disability, gender, sexuality, religion, or language understand citizenship as more. It is the embodiment of freedom and belonging, the responsibility of being an integral part of the whole, and the active engagement in our collective future.

If we thought of politics as a system through which we take care of each other and the whole of society, then citizenship would be the practice of taking care of each other. This understanding of politics and citizenship would mean getting educated about the issues that matter. It would mean having courageous conversations with our peers about oppression and inequality. It would mean organizing around values of collective care and ensuring that no one gets left behind. It would mean voting for candidates who reflect our values and running for office ourselves. And it would mean repairing the wounds of our past and detoxifying ourselves of the myths of separation, scarcity, and supremacy. The practice of citizenship is how we uphold the freedom and dignity of everyone and achieve collective well-being for all. It's loving and fighting for all of us, not just some of us. And it's actively cocreating a future where everyone can thrive.

Well-being is only possible with the full participation and realization of all of its parts. And many of us are catching on to the "inconvenient truth" that we are not separate from the suffering of all people and the planet. We're now seeing the very real implications of the history of extraction and exploitation that has gotten us here. And the truth is, it won't get us much further. We are staring down the end of times, and unless we do something different, we are facing our own extinction. The only way forward is to confront anything and everything that is in the way of our collective well-being and build a new future where every single one of us belongs and has what we need to thrive.

PERSONAL INQUIRY

I know that to heal I must return to myself over and over and over again. I learn to sit with my fear and longing with curiosity and compassion. I give thanks for how it may have served me when I needed it most. I let go of the ways it may no longer be serving me. I belong to my stories but I am not them. I belong to my mistakes but I am not them. I belong to myself first and foremost but not solely. As I breathe down deeply into my roots that weave and tangle with other roots, I can feel myself as something bigger than myself. I belong to you. We belong to each other.

- In what places, activities, and people do you feel a deep sense of belonging?
- What are the stories you were taught about what it means to be American?
- How does your social location inform whose struggles you feel drawn to engage with and whose struggles you feel indifferent to?
- What role has fear played in preventing you from showing up and advocating for the well-being of everyone?
- What are some ways in your life you can move from othering to bridging?
- What is one thing that you can do every day as a citizen who is committed to the well-being of everyone?

Building a Future of Belonging

I remember in the immediate aftermath of 9/11, before the dust had settled, before we got afraid, there was this opening. In that space, there was no certainty, no safety, no handbook for how to respond—there was just *us*. All of us, stunned, heartbroken, and awake. And we did the only thing we knew to do—we turned toward one another. We gave blood, we made casseroles, we planted flowers. It was not the kind of patriotism that places our love for our country above our love for one another. There is nothing un-American about asking hard questions about how we got here, what's in the way of well-being, who's missing, and how we can all thrive. Parallel to our history of oppression is a history of resilience that courses through our veins. Our ancestors have passed down a spirit of resistance that has survived enormous challenges in the long arc toward justice and well-being. Their persistence is our strength as we continue the work and become the ancestors of our future.

The story of 9/11 that we don't hear about as much was one that emerged on stairwells, in kitchens, and at bodegas. It is the story of a citizenship awakened, unified in solidarity and survival in the face of the unimaginable. Thousands converged at the site with only a desire to be of service, but many quickly found purpose. There were those who would become known as the Bucket Brigade, a mass assembly line of people who carried debris to investigators so they could search for human remains. There were calls for supplies—boots, sweatshirts, cigarettes, Gatorade, whatever—that flooded into makeshift drop-off sites in lower Manhattan. Countless trays of lasagna and casseroles flowed into the homes of survivors and volunteer food stations. Half a million people donated blood, more than was needed, as there were only survivors and the dead and little in between. Priests, ministers, and monks showed up simply to listen and offer spiritual comfort. There were singers and artists, strangers and neighbors who simply found a way to make a meaningful contribution. All of it under the radar and self-organized by people who felt compelled to act.

In *A Paradise Built in Hell*, Rebecca Solnit captures the spirit of reconnection that follows a crisis.[34] She chronicles the events that came after the 1906 earthquake in San Francisco, Hurricane Katrina, 9/11, and others and examines human resilience in times of crisis. What she finds in her research is that disasters don't just destroy, they create. They bring out the best in humanity—not a relentless instinct to defend and survive, but a community spirit that is almost contagious. In the aftermath of these disasters were random acts of kindness, deep altruism, unparalleled cooperation, a renewed civic temperament, even joy. Yes, joy. "Joy doesn't betray but sustains activism," writes Solnit.[35] It becomes an opportunity for people to see how good life can be when the system breaks down and it's no longer business as usual. "If paradise now arises in hell, it is because in the suspension of the usual order and the failure of most systems, we are free to live and act another way."[36] And it is in the breakdown—in the falling apart of structures and the dismantling of systems—that healing can emerge. We find ourselves in those spaces—the parts of us that are resilient and creative and subversive—and we remember that we have the power to transform ourselves and one another.

Organizing is how we take care of each other. And it starts where we are. What begins at the local level expands, so that our efforts and resources aggregate for love and justice. We move on behalf of the whole (not the few) in collective action with social and political movements that advance our values and democratize well-being for all. This requires both organizing depth (in how we build trust/relationships and create culture) and scale (in how we engage the disengaged and bridge across movements). It is a holistic approach to organizing through personal practice, community building, and collective action as we transform ourselves and restructure our world to support the conditions of well-being for all.

We the people are the heart of this ecology, and what we believe about ourselves and one another matters. Together we must reclaim our power as citizens and build a capacity to be active creators and stewards of our communities. For centuries, institutions have told people (especially marginalized people) that they don't have power, that they must settle for the status quo and accept the reality we are living in. But nonviolence and restorative justice trainer Kazu Haga reminds us that we have to "cut through the delusion that we are powerless" and realize that together we have the power to change our conditions.[37] Organizing is just that: it creates the conditions where more people have the power to resist and create systems that take care of everyone. It is the unofficial fourth branch of our government, "we the people," that exercises our collective political power to influence a politics of well-being that takes care of everyone.

Building political power around values of well-being is not about unity over difference. It's about building a coalition that centers and celebrates difference. The only way to win—and by win I mean to actually end the "imperialist white supremacist capitalist patriarchy" as bell hooks describes it[38]—is to unleash the power of our diversity and build across lines of difference.* It means centering the leadership and perspectives of the most marginalized to build a radically inclusive movement for all. The Combahee River Collective understood this when they saw "black feminism as the logical political movement to combat the manifold and simultaneous oppressions that all women of color face." They went on to say that "if black women were free, it would mean that everyone else was free since our freedom would necessitate the destruction of all systems of oppression."[39] The intersectional foundations laid by the Combahee River Collective encourage us to identify the common ground on which to make coalition possible across profound cultural, racial, class, sex, gender, and power differences. From there, we can build a politics of well-being that breaks from our oppressive roots *and* embraces the complexity and potential of our many lived experiences as the way we get free together.

It took the sky falling and the ground breaking on 9/11 for me to wake up. And it gave me a glimpse of who we can become when we rise to the occasion. Which makes me wonder: What kind of future will we be confronted with as conflict continues and climate change ravages our planet? And who will we be when that moment arrives? Better yet, who will we be today and tomorrow? We don't need another crisis to wake us up. We don't need to be knocked down and torn apart to reclaim our agency and collective will. We don't need to be betrayed by the system to realize it is a lie. We don't need catastrophic loss to remember the sacredness of all life.

Grace Lee Boggs reminds us that visionary organizing "begin[s by] creating images and stories of the future that help us imagine and create alternatives to the existing system."[40] It is an invitation to imagine better and tell a new story of who "we" are—the big we—so that we forge a new path that is rooted in interdependence, regeneration, and mutuality. We must, as Dr.

---

* With over thirty works, bell hooks has written some of the most influential books on feminism, race, and love. Here are some must-reads: *Ain't I a Woman?*, *All About Love*, *Feminism Is for Everybody*, *Where We Stand: Class Matters*, and *Killing Rage: Ending Racism*.

King encouraged us, "undergo a radical revolution of values . . . We must rapidly begin to shift from a 'thing-oriented' society to a 'person-oriented' society."[41] When we can align and act from these values, we can build new futures of possibility and potential. We can take our place in the world and do our part to create the conditions of collective care and well-being. And despite the wounds of our past and the reality of our present, we can still have hope. "To hope is to gamble," Rebecca Solnit says. "It's to bet on the future, on your desires, on the possibility that an open heart and uncertainty is better than gloom and safety. To hope is dangerous, and yet it is the opposite of fear, for to live is to risk."[42]

COLLECTIVE PRACTICE: BUILD COLLECTIVE POWER

We the people have the power to change our circumstances and shape our collective future. It starts with choosing to be together differently and actively engaging in self-governance. #WeGovern defines *governance* as "the process by which people determine the norms and rules that guide people's everyday life and behavior."[43] It is how we choose to live together and take care of the shared home that we call Earth. It is how we protect and uphold one another's well-being. It is how we share resources and create the conditions for everyone to thrive. It is how we respond to harm and advocate for change and accountability. And it is how we reimagine and build new systems and structures that reflect our values and take care of everyone.

Organizing reveals the power of ordinary people to do extraordinary things together. In small groups of shared practice and ongoing relationships, we grow in our depth of commitment and our ability to take action. These circles (also known as pods, squads, small groups) are the vehicle of our movement. They are not structures of transaction but structures of trust that build our capacity to meet each moment and respond with courage and care. They also are a means for expressing our diversity, agency, and creativity to respond to local needs, addressing varying issues, or representing different communities. Whether we are coming together to build climate resilience, to protect each other, to create mutual aid, or to do anti-racism work, circles reveal our shared potential and power. Circles start small to enable us to be agile and adaptive, intimate and relational in response to the many crises we are facing. But they have the potential to replicate and aggregate around the country, demonstrating our collective power in reach, scale, and impact. In this final practice of our journey together, the invitation is to circle up and discover the power you have to show up and build the future that we all deserve.

1. Find your people: This is a process of mapping and reflection about who is in your network, what is needed, and how you can come together. It could be a gathering of your neighborhood block, your peers and colleagues, your friends and family, or anyone with whom you share values or a commitment to change.*

2. Circle up: Invite three or more friends, peers, or neighbors to gather together for your first meeting. Consider the space (whether in-person or virtual) to

---

* The Bay Area Transformative Justice Collective suggests using the term *pod* to describe the kind of relationship between people who turn to each other around ongoing safety, accountability, and transformation of behaviors, or individual and collective healing and resiliency. Here's a helpful pod-mapping tool: https://batjc .wordpress.com/resources/pods-and-pod-mapping-worksheet/.

ensure people feel supported and welcome in the environment. Invite folks to make a contribution to the experience through the sharing of food, music, poetry, meditation, and more.

3. Build culture: Discuss the values, assumptions, and agreements you will center and practice together. Cocreating the conditions in this way not only fosters trust and relationship building, but it also helps us build a capacity to hold conflict and change when it arises.

4. Determine your purpose: Explore what and how you want to learn together or work together or grow together. What are the needs in your community? What resources do you have access to? What are the goals of your pod? What else?

5. Practice cooperation and accountability: Be sure to make space for everyone's input. How you embrace group decision-making and accountability is a reflection of how you show up for each other.

6. Locate yourself in the larger movement: Consider where you fit into your community and how your group can support and be in support and solidarity with other groups in the wider movement.

CHAPTER 8

Reimagining Wellness

There are those who want the world to remain on its current path. This is not only unacceptable, it is painfully unimaginative. For the beauty of our generation is we are uniquely situated to achieve what so many in this world currently consider impossible. How exquisitely beautiful it will be to watch the current narrative go down in flames, then witness poetics & phoenix rise from the ashes.

Embers, ancestors and angels await us loved ones. Forward.

MARK GONZALES

The lessons of our interdependence are coming at us fast and have a clear message for us: either we reckon with the past or we risk the future. Some are likening it to an apocalypse. While the term *apocalypse* often refers to the complete and final destruction of the world (as described in the Bible's book of Revelation), the etymology of the word actually means "to uncover or reveal." This moment is not just an unraveling but an unveiling of the truths and medicine that have always been here. Thriving in the face of this will demand a commitment and capacity that none of us can muster on our own. We will need the depth of our courage and the width of our connections if we stand a chance against extreme inequality, mutating pandemics, climate calamity, and mass migration. We must reach outside ourselves, across divides, beyond borders, and toward one another—not just to ensure our collective survival but to realize our full potential.

"We are in an imagination battle," says adrienne maree brown.[1] Imagination enabled people to buy into the idea that they are entitled to someone else's land or that anyone can achieve the American Dream or that we can police one another into safety. Imagination inspired people to pursue the perfect human race or a magic pill for well-being and enlightenment. Imagination created nation states and built walls that separated who is in and who is out. And imagination made it possible to enslave and exploit humans for the sake of greed and power. This sort of imagination was shaped by ideologies of separation, scarcity, and supremacy. For years I bought into this story, contorting myself to fit into someone else's dream. Not only is the story limiting, but it is violent and harmful, and if we don't reimagine what is possible, it is going to lead us to more wars, wildfires, pandemics, and eventually extinction. Building the wellness that we all deserve is both a remembering and a reimagining of what's possible.

We need only look to nature for how to survive an apocalypse. Nature understands our interdependence. Take the body, for example. There is not one system of the body that can survive without the other interconnected systems. If a part of the body—an organ, a cell—is in need of aid, another part of the body responds with energy, nutrients, oxygen, or the removal of wastes to repair the body and restore it to balance. Everything works in relationship to ensure the well-being of the whole. Nature affirms that the legacy of separation and supremacy that we have inherited is not only unnatural but deadly. And it shows us that the path to collective healing and well-being is to build a diverse and life-affirming ecosystem that understands the value of all of its parts.

We are all first responders on the front lines of our shared future. But our work will look different based on our location. We must ask ourselves "What is my role in the revolution?" and remember that we are not the first and we are not alone. As we build the future that we all deserve, we must "follow the Ones who know The Way," as movement strategist Taj James reminds us.[2] Those at the periphery have the clearest view and vision of the whole system—of what is broken and who's been broken by it, of what is needed and how. When we listen closely to those who are most exposed and impacted by society's ills, we can best respond with creative solutions for our collective survival.

So on this last leg of our journey, I've turned to the wisdom and experience of those who know—those who are working to reach beyond dominant paradigms of "normal," break the molds of white supremacy, capitalism, and individualism, and live into ways of being that heal the wounds that are holding us back and imagine new practices and structures that take care of everyone. I invited six people who are working across different intersections to share how we can create more possibilities for a future of well-being that works for everyone.

Norma Wong (Norma Ryuko Kawelokū Wong Roshi) is a teacher at the Institute of Zen Studies and Daihonzan Chozen-ji, having trained in Zen for nearly forty years. She works as a thought and strategy partner to community and justice activists. **Anasa Troutman** is cultural strategist, writer, producer, developer, philanthropist, and impact investor. As founder and CEO of The BIG We and executive director of Historic Clayborn Temple, Anasa works in community with artists, entrepreneurs, and capital stewards to invest in emerging leaders, heal our culture, and cocreate a world of joy, abundance, and love for all. **Mark Gonzales** is a futurist; he develops tools, tech, and narratives to ignite civic imagination and shape human existence. He is the chair of the Department of the Future and a 2019/2020 Kennedy Center Fellow of the Citizen Arts. **Teo Drake** is a spiritual activist, an educator, a practicing Buddhist and yogi, and an artisan who works in wood and steel. A blue-collar, queer trans man living with AIDS, Teo is an activist at the intersections of gender, sexuality, race, class, ability, and spirituality. **Taj James** is a father, poet, strategist, ecosystem designer, and capital advisor. Working with transformational leaders, small teams, networks, and anchor institutions, Taj enjoys exploring what it means to nurture the community we have and create the community we need. **Dr.**

Jasmine Syedullah is a black feminist political theorist of abolition, as well as coauthor of *Radical Dharma: Talking Race, Love, and Liberation*. She is an assistant professor in Vassar College's Africana Studies Program.

In our conversation, I asked questions about what is in the way of our collective well-being and how we can get there. A number of shared themes emerged that speak to what collective wellness looks like in practice including remembering who we are, how we "be" together, practicing accountability, creating a culture of care, building the future by repairing the past, and creating a just and joyful transition. Their words provide direction in an uncertain moment and hope amid despair. And what emerges in the collective weaving of their stories and wisdom reveals possibility—and that we are much closer than we are far apart.

As Arundhati Roy has said, the disruption caused by the COVID-19 pandemic and other such moments of reckoning "is a portal, a gateway between one world and the next. We can choose to walk through it, dragging the carcasses of our prejudice and hatred, our avarice, our data banks and dead ideas, our dead rivers and smoky skies behind us. Or we can walk through lightly, with little luggage, ready to imagine another world. And ready to fight for it."[3] This conversation is about how we show up for this moment and move toward the more joyful and liberated world we are all yearning for.

KERRI KELLY: *This book examines the myths and lies that are holding us back and making us unwell. What do we need to reclaim and remember in order to heal forward?*

TAJ JAMES: *Around 5,000 years ago or so, an idea emerged in human history that no one had ever thought of before, which was just this notion that as human beings, we are not a part of nature, we are separate from nature. And we're not just separate, we are separate and above. We are separate and superior. And so that notion of that story, that idea, that cultural narrative, that human beings are separate from nature, which is spiritually, biologically, materially in every way, a lie, became the basis of how human societies reorganize themselves.*

We've forgotten who we are. And the simple solution is to remember who we are. I love that Harry Belafonte song "Turn the World Around"—"Do I know who I am, do I know who you are, do we see each other clearly, do we know who we are?" And no, we don't. We don't, we don't, we don't. The great turning, the great awakening, the great return is to just remember who we are and to honor, and defend, and protect the sacred, and all of our relations. It's a simple process.

The other aspect of that lie as it has emerged is we've disconnected ourselves from the web of life and we've also disconnected ourselves generationally. We think about what a person is as the thing that is born and the thing that dies—as opposed to knowing that we are embodiments of multigenerational arcs with responsibilities to our ancestors and to our descendants. We are our ancestors and we are our descendants, in every way that you can imagine. So the other aspect of remembering who we are is reclaiming our place in our multigenerational arc. Seven generations back, and seven generations forward, living in that arc of sacred responsibility. That remembering would change everything about how we do everything. That remembering, that awakening, is underway.

Roshi Norma Wong: *We've somehow forgotten how to practice in a way in which we hold a discipline of constant evolution. It's here and then, rather than here and now. In the Buddhist context, the here and now is immediately replaced by another here and now. It's so instantaneous that the consciousness that you have to have to always hold on to the new now, we'd say that's the energy that you need for a just transition. It's that you're part of the whole. In other words, even though you're coming into the new now, you hold everything that happened in the past, including everything that you remember and don't remember. And the paradox is, if you are in your total consciousness around what has to happen right now, you prepare in entirety for the future. And you begin to remember the past in more granular detail, but there's also a way in which it isn't a rupture. So you remember the past when you have the capacity to remember it. That's when you truly remember it.*

So when the bones of Indigenous children come out of the ground at a boarding school in a province in Canada, the bones are coming above the ground because we can now embrace those ancestors. We can now actually remember them; we don't need to shut them out. We don't need to have it be something that we set aside. We now have the capacity to do that, and that's why they're

229

being made known to us at that point in time. And while they're not, they stay safely within ground. So the long-forgottenness that we have means that that is our prevalent habit pattern.

TAJ: *There are cultures and traditions that have not forgotten, that are here helping remind the rest of us who have forgotten how to find our way back home, back into the web of life, and back into our intergenerational arc of responsibility. Not a moment too soon, because the world built around the lie of separation and supremacy is fundamentally in crisis. And so now we have to figure out how to remember who we are, to care for each other, to care for the water, and to welcome the stranger, and to help those who are in motion. Because we've so destabilized the globe—politically, culturally, economically, and climate-wise—that we're looking at really unprecedented levels of human migration. As the floods flow, and the fires burn, and the seas rise, and the crops burn on the vine with extreme heat, and parts of the world are just becoming too hot for human beings to live in, there's going to be a lot of people in motion. But what is essential is that, even with all of the violence and harm we've done to Mother Earth and the web of life, there is still so much abundance. Mother Earth is still so generous; there's still, in the midst of all of that destruction and pain, more than enough for all of us to thrive. If we honor each other, and figure out ways to take care of each other, and make sure everyone has what they need, there's still more than enough. Even with all of the destruction that this lie and the systems built around it have wrought. That's the good news.*

KERRI: *The dominant wellness culture is deeply rooted in toxic individualism and the glorification of the "small self" at the expense of the "big we." How do we move from a wellness of me to a wellness of we?*

ANASA TROUTMAN: *The honest truth is that the wellness of we requires the wellness of me. And so many of us are not well, we are pretending, pretending, pretending so hard. The irony is that there is no path to the we but through the me, but you have to really do that in a real way. Egoically, it doesn't mean making a show, it means actually being committed to your wellness, which means that you realize that you are a part of the sacred circle of life and that you're not in there by yourself. And the things that you do matter, they actually matter. And you cannot be wantonly violent or wantonly patriarchal or wantonly white supremacist, regardless of your race or age or ability or sexual orientation or gender or anything else. We all have the capacity to harm each other based on these tropes that are out of alignment with what is true spirit. And unless we can see the dichotomy of who we are as individuals and who we are as a collective and act accordingly, as if the whole is the self and the self is the whole, then these things that you're asking for are not possible.*

Even with all of the advances that we've made socially and through civics and laws and morality, fundamentally we still are in a place that believes that if you are a wealthy, heterosexual, cisgender, white man, then your life is more valuable. Because if you have more access, more tools, you have more. So there's no accounting for collective wellness. It's not going to happen. And it doesn't matter what we do on a small scale—the tactics are not going to get us to the larger shift. It doesn't matter how much money people donate or how many kids you put in a program or whatever. If we want fundamental shifts, we have to make fundamental shifts. And those ways that we approach change right now are not fundamental, they're tactical. We are climbing molehills and not seeing vistas. That's just the truth of the matter.

We have unwell community practices, unwell personal practices, unwell legislation, unwell everything because our culture is unwell, so that begs the question, What does a well culture look like and how do we get there? The only way for us to get where we're going is for our culture to be well and for the very foundation of society to be fertilized with something else, so we can grow different things. That's basic biomimicry. In chemistry class, if you want to grow something in the petri dish, you put one kind of culture in it. If you want to grow something else, you have to change the culture at the bottom of the petri dish so you can facilitate the growth of something new. So if we want to facilitate the growth of an equitable, well society, we have to feed it with something different. And the question that I keep bumping up against is, Do we have the capacity to actually change our very fundamental way of being so that we can grow something new?

TEO DRAKE: *Really embracing nonduality is a big part of this, because dominant culture and dominant wellness culture are so hierarchical, leading us to think this step needs to be achieved before we can take the next step. Even yoga poses get talked about this way—beginner, intermediate, advanced, etc. But living and loving and existing and healing and getting well within communities that are devalued and targets of oppression means being able to really hold, through vulnerability and heartbreak, the inseparable truths that I need my people to survive and at the same time my community needs me to survive. I will do just about anything to ensure that my people will survive, but part of wrestling with self-worth is simultaneously embracing that my communities need me to survive.*

And in order for me to survive I have to allow others to participate in my well-being and my healing as I am participating in my own healing and in the healing of others—other individuals and the collective whole. That can happen in the ebb and flow of attention—sometimes I need to attend a bit more to what's happening to me, sometimes my attention is a bit more focused outwardly on others—but they never exist outside of that both/and. So the nonduality—the both/and—is how we break down the false dichotomy of me/we. I don't need either of those to dissolve; I need to understand that they are of one another.

And yes, there's a dominant culture of wellness, but there's also generations and generations of nondominant cultures of well-being. We don't have to be at war with something that's not working and that's harming us; we can just put it down and turn toward wisdom and ways of healing. I am always deeply suspicious of anything that tries to pull me out of connection with myself and with others. Instead, I turn toward ways of being and healing and working that call me home to myself and call me home to belonging.

KERRI: *How do we work together—with the understanding that we are impacted in different and disproportionate ways—to build a future of well-being for all?*

JASMINE SYEDULLAH: *A lot of folks are encouraging us to get out of our comfort zones in terms of anti-racism and disability justice, saying that if you talk to people who are different from you and create relationships, then it'll be better. And I kind of agree, but I also think there might be a little bit more to that protocol than just cornering some people who don't have time for you and hoping for the best, right? It's not just about building relationships with people, it's about* building ethical relationships. *Relationships of mutual thriving, growth, and care can literally change the quality of our collective consciousness. Having the humility to face the truth of multiple consciousnesses that you wouldn't have access to otherwise begins with a conversation. Sometimes the conversation can change your own consciousness, but in my experience, a conversation isn't enough. We need books. We need poetry. We need film. We need multiple points of contact. Shifts in consciousness exist at the convergence of multiple encounters with difference. And it's not fair to put all of your consciousness-raising on the generosity of one buddy who is experiencing the world differently from you. That's a lot to put on an individual.*

ANASA: *I often say, "Don't talk to me about diversity and equity. Just be honest, just tell the truth." Because the truth has yet to be told. And if relationships are required as a first but meaningful step towards equity, and the relationship is not built on transparency, vulnerability, honesty, and trust, then it's not a real relationship—and it's not going to be a bridge to anything except more brokenness and more deceit and more violation. And the first, most major problem we have is that the culture that has us deny the sacred nature of our life is also the culture that has not equipped us to have meaningful, open, tender, difficult conversations. And most of the folks who need to be in the conversation frankly are not equipped to be in the conversation.*

And I don't mean just white people. All of us have difficulty with what is required for those kinds of conversations—courage and transparency and vulnerability and honesty, but also grace and the ability to weep together and to not have answers, because who knows what the answer is? Can we just all sit down and be like, "Nobody in here knows what the fuck we're going to do. We know where we are and we know where we want to go, but none of us know how to get there." Let's just start there, because that's the truth. We all have ideas and we all have leanings and we all have things that we are compelled to do and things that we are doing and working on to some degree, but nobody knows how to get to the point where we actually can have wellness for all people. And until and unless we can collectively get to the point where we can have that conversation, I don't see how we're going to do anything but have incremental legislated change.

ROSHI NORMA: *If you cut through the habit of the political construct and go to the practical factual and spirit ways of indigeneity, you come close to the worldview of what it would mean if we remembered as people that are on the same island. Islands have mothers in a modern context, so it's not about returning to old ways. It's about returning to a different relationship with other beings, known and unknown, loved and unloved, humans and not. And then, figuring out the really complex ways in which you would then have to live if that were the case. If you have mutuality, then an argument cannot be carried out by stakeholders. This—whatever this issue is—is not about balancing the needs of stakeholders. It is about figuring out what all of the stewards require. If you are in this—not as a person who is a stakeholder, but you're in here as a steward—then the mutuality of what you need to come to would have to work out in a different way because, among other things, your governance is not a matter of a hierarchical governance. Other people have to figure it out, and then we are the people who have to carry it out. We are the people who will need to live in it. And we are the people who are responsible that the next generation and the generation after continue to carry out the stewardship of whatever this mutual responsibility, the sacred responsibility, happens to be.*

JASMINE: *Work that brings us to our knees in reverence to those whose lives we don't understand is absolutely fundamental and necessary in order for us to change what we're producing right now, which is isolation and siloing and schism and separation. And the way we do that is really by honoring the knowledge of those who are different from us. If you don't come from a tradition that really knows how to honor, that's also something to notice and acknowledge. And recognize that you actually need to watch and learn what reverence looks like, and feels like, from others generous enough to model it. Learn how to practice reverence in a way that has integrity with who you are and meets you where you're at.*

We've got to be like: "Oh, you know what? The way that I've been doing things, thinking that I know everything and thinking that I control the outcome and thinking that I can figure it all out through science or technology or something, is inadequate. What I actually need is your witness. What I actually need is your experience. What I actually need is to kneel at the altar of what

234

you know. Not so I can take it all for myself, but so that we can work together, because I'll never know what you know, right? But if we work together, then we can work with what we both know and figure out another way to move together through the experience of trauma, through the experience of grief, through the experience of triumph in ways that aren't competitive but rather complement one another's strengths." This is what we mean in radical dharma when we talk about the framework for liberation. The framework has five aspects or pillars, and the fifth is collective process. So much of the way we organize collectivity is based on models of power that reinforce hierarchies of power and privilege we have been conditioned to accept and believe are inescapable. A radical dharma of collective process honors what each individual brings to the table—not just their personal skills and passion, but also their people, protocols, practices, and imaginations for the future.

KERRI: *Accountability is often viewed as bad or shameful, something to be avoided or deflected. How can we change our relationship to accountability as something that is necessary for building community?*

MARK GONZALES: *We have to acknowledge that our social understanding of justice and accountability have been overwhelmingly shaped by a pop culture of shoot-'em-up films, it-all-works-out-in-the-end web series, imprisonment headlines, and more. As such, when many of us say the word* accountability, *what we really mean is* vengeance. *By no means am I saying let's jump from vengeance to forgive-and-forget models that perpetuate harm, especially when imposed upon individuals by external arbitrators with little or no input from those being harmed. What I am asking us to realize is that as we build new systems for governing relationships in society, to anticipate that justice will look different, not by society and culture, but by individuals as well. We are all well aware in the well-being field—as well as the medical field—of the concept "different people need different medicine." Why is it so hard for us to fathom then that we will need different forms of justice as well? Isn't justice, at its best, meant to be a form of medicine?*

This is why I believe grace and accountability are what we need more of in our decision-making process. Without grace, we are building a pitfall at the end of our current decision-making processes, where we all fall to the pitchforks.

Without accountability, we only ask for forgiveness, appealing to the better angels, instead of challenging us to become them. With these two elements, our mindset shifts from disposable and punitive, to course-corrective and karmic. The two core elements that guide a regenerative system that we talk so much about and truly desire but have yet to see at scale.

JASMINE: *We are reproducing the conditions of our own insecurities by relying on a punitive practice of accountability. We are. A lot of times, people who have questions about abolition ask, "What are we going to do with the murderers and the rapists?" And I say, "One thing I can tell you for sure is that the system, as it exists, is creating more murderers and rapists than anywhere else in the world." But of course we're terrified of those things because we don't realize that the punitive correction system that we're relying on is mass-producing them. That is what it produces. And I'm not just talking about people that get locked up. I'm talking about the people who do the locking up. I'm talking about the people who do the policing. I'm talking about the people who are judges. We're actually creating more violence in our societies by taking people away from their families, by subjecting people to dehumanizing technologies of torture that they not only have to be targeted by, but also that they have to maintain. Meeting correction officers, police officers, with these high rates of depression, high rates of suicide—never mind domestic violence and the ways that we internalize that and turn it out towards other people. This is a system that produces insecurity. And so wellness, health, security, safety all rely on figuring out a different way. A different way to hold each other accountable that doesn't rely on punitive retaliation and torture and violence to create safety.*

Accountability as wellness helps us affirm every stage of the process of coming into consciousness, choice, integrity, and repair. This comes up a lot in the classroom for me. What I've noticed in myself and in my students is that we are so afraid of failure, right? We don't want to get a bad grade. We don't want to not know something. We don't want to get something wrong. This comes up a lot with white students in conversations about race. They say, "It's not my place" and "I don't want to make a mistake" and "I also don't want to get it wrong." But accountability looks like learning to love up on our mistakes, our failures, the ways that we fall short—not showing up with everything prepped and ready.

So I see accountability as an existential imperative but also as play, as satire. If we can't laugh at ourselves and how awkward it is to learn to be a decent human being, then we risk endlessly reproducing the punitive relationship to belonging we set out to resist! One of the questions I bring to the students I teach is: How can we be in touch with and present with the ways that we fail and embrace them with curiosity, bring a sense of humor in to bear witness to ourselves and each other in ways that create more room for iteration, improvisation, and improvement, for trying again. How might we come to see accountability as a practice we can learn from rather than a performance we have to nail in order to win—a practice in becoming more accountable to each other in our fullness in real time. The reality is that each of us has hurt people. And some of that hurt is our responsibility. It would be great if we didn't hold our responsibility for harm with so much shame and shutdown and punishment that we can't connect to the invitations they contain to teach us more about ourselves.

ANASA: *In a culture of wellness, accountability is care. In a culture of extraction, accountability is violence. That fundamental shift has to be made, and it can only be made in pockets. Because it's not something that you can legislate or mandate. If you can't mandate a frigging mask, you can't mandate someone being comfortable with being held accountable. So it has to happen in communities. It's a decision that we have to make every day. Because we have to practice it. It's messy and hard and painful until it's not, until it's just like, "Oh right, you're right, girl, I'm sorry. You're right. I won't do that again." When you have a practice of accountability with someone else, after a certain amount of time, the transparency, the lovingly calling out, the correction and the apology happens in the moment. When you don't have that, it could take a lifetime, if it ever happens. And so relationships cannot happen without accountability. And accountability is required for a relationship to actually be authentic and for it to be a bridge to go literally anywhere.*

KERRI: *The many crises of this moment are a culmination of the wounds of the past gone unacknowledged and unattended. How do we build a future from this place?*

Roshi Norma: *There's a good amount of both individual and collective healing that would need to occur. You could do a whole chapter on what healing is and what healing isn't, right? I think that "healing" is not used with enough gravity in the ways in which we speak the word. When I talk to people about their restoration of their humanity, there's a part where you can get trapped in a place that is only about one's survival. But you should not conflate that part of you that's in survival as being healed. You're just in survival. And the way that your cellular memory works—both your physical cellular memory and your spiritual cellular memory—is that if you are in survival for too long a time period, you begin to actually think of that as the norm. And survival is a state of survival and not a state of thriving.*

So you would say the entire world is in a collective trauma, of which we are just in various stages and in different stories around that. And if that is the case, irrespective of whether you are a bad actor or a good actor or a bystander, essentially we're just all in this collective trauma. It's taken thousands of years for us to get to this point. And so, whatever your political ideology may be in that regard, political wins and losses will come and go. Whether or not humanity will make the turn is a much longer and consequential process.

Taj: *You have to repair the harm of the past if you're going to have any hope of creating a regenerative economic future. Why do white people not want to do that? Why do people want to skip over the work of repair, and just skip on to the clean-tech, green, regenerative future? Because there's often a sense of responsibility for past harms that people don't want to account for, for all kinds of reasons. In the work of a transition from an extractive economy to a regenerative economy, we have to center the work of reparations, repair, and land back as the driver of the transition into our regenerative future. We have to account for and reckon with how we got here. If we don't acknowledge the harms of the past, we're going to reproduce the thinking that created the harm and create some new eco-apartheid future.*

Jasmine: *We have to reckon with the harms that have been done in our name, in the places that we call home in a collective way, and create healing around that. We can figure it out. There's a ton of resources for truth and reconciliation, for reparative practices, for transformative justice. We kind of got that. What we don't have are practices for reckoning with the past and dealing with past harm and collective culpability. For example, I'm in the academy and everyone's doing land acknowledgments. What would it mean for land acknowledgments to be more than performative or more than perfunctory or more than checking the box? What would an action-based acknowledgment look like? And for institutions like mine that have admitted to and been found out for housing the bones of Indigenous people in basements and closets without ceremony and without integrity, what does apology look like? What does acknowledgment look like then?*

To me, that looks like the future. Acknowledging the past, recognizing the violence and harm that has been done, and then paying it forward by, for example, dedicating part of an endowment to an ongoing program of free tuition for Native students who can get into the school. Creating a fund where they can come for free for the next fifty generations. An abolitionist future requires that we be willing to be changed, as Mary Hooks of Southerners on New Ground proclaims in her mandate "in service to the work." And by allowing ourselves transformation we create space for the transformation of stale and outmoded aspects of our collective consciousness.

TAJ: *It's essential that we don't reproduce binary ways as we work to transcend the binaries that are killing us. We have to do the spiritual work, and the cultural work, and the healing work of releasing ourselves from the binary worldview and the binary story that says some of us are above and some of us are below, and some of us are good and some of us are bad, and you just have to figure out which one you are and play your role appropriately. There's no way out of the binary mess if we just reproduce the binary way. So the first task is to just remember who we are. The binary is a lie. We have to embrace contradictions so that we can navigate living in simultaneity. Because past, present, and future are one. In some ways that appears to be a paradox, but it's actually just the nature of reality. Past, present, and future are one. We carry the past with us, we carry the future with us. We have responsibility to the past, we have responsibility to the future. It's a very, very practical truth. In some ways it's esoteric, but in every way it is more real than the chair that I'm sitting in. So we've got to get real. We are essentially living simultaneously in a collapsing past and in an emergent future. And we are the physical bridge and embodiments, carrying the energy from the past into the future.*

KERRI: *Many people are waking up to the fact that the culture of domination and extraction we've inherited is not only threatening our individual and collective well-being, but it's threatening our survival. But what exactly is the world we are trying to build?*

TEO: *I think the notion that we're trying to make something that does not yet exist actually does a disservice to the many threads of a new world that have been and are being nurtured and built. There are communities who are living out wisdom that can serve all of us. I do believe we need, wholesale, a radical change. At the same time we need to honor the seeds of the new world that exist in these current conditions. We need to practice awe and reverence for the fact that people have the courage and audacity to live with one another in ways that completely defy the undervaluing of that way of being.*

I see it all the time in the ways that those of us whom society has deemed disposable refuse to be disposed. The ways that people stop asking the uncaring oppressive powers that be for crumbs and turn toward one another instead. The ways that people create underground economies, create networks of care, craft policies—without law degrees—that make communities safe. I see evidence of it all the time. Building this new world is a big undertaking, and it's already in motion. If it can happen in the most hostile and least welcoming of environments, it can flourish if we change the conditions. That's where hope lies for me. That's the hill that cynicism dies on. If it can happen in these harsh conditions, imagine what can happen if we turn our hope and our hearts and our will toward it.

ANASA: *The future of well-being and collective care is alive in my own community here in Memphis. The way that people relate to and take care of themselves and each other is transforming in such a profound way. It's happening all over the country though, and I can't attest to it but most likely it's happening all over the world. The collective is transforming. We are being pulled towards the "big we." For those of us who have already been in these conversations, the pull towards it is irresistible, and some who were indifferent before are becoming curious and wondering what it would take for our collective wellness to take hold. Lots of community groups, artist circles, especially after COVID and the uprising of 2020, so many examples of people who live in community on the same block taking turns cooking for and feeding each other, groups and organizations who have made the commitment to not bring the police in when harm is done in their communities, and learning how to employ community-centered public health and safety models, families making the choice to educate and nurture their children together. It's happening. With patience, diligence, and tenacity, it's happening.*

TAJ: *Our friends at Movement Generation remind us that, in the Western tradition, the root of the word* economy *is* eco, *and* eco *means home, and* economy *means basically the management of home. And so, if the economy is just about managing home, then how well are we doing taking care of home? Home is the place where we should be safe, and where we get our needs met, and where we figure out how we take care of each other. The experience of the economy over the last 500 to 5,000 years is that we take care of each other within hierarchies and binaries. And we place some things above other things, and the things that are above dominate the things that are below. We've been taking care of home through strategies of violence, domination, and control, in which some groups concentrate power in order to control other groups, in order to reproduce society. But there are also ways to organize society that are based on interdependence, interbeing, cooperation, care, and not violence, domination, and extraction.*

The question of economies is the question of the quality of our relationships. What are the values that are embedded in how our relationships are organized? Our relationships of care, production, reproduction. To think about the economy holistically, we have to think in a different way: energy is energy, water is water, capital is energy that needs to flow like water. The difference between ice and water and steam—it's just water. Money is just another form of energy. And the question is, How have we organized it? We've created mechanisms to extract energy out of people and the environment, in ways that are violent, harmful, and unsustainable. What if we thought about how we organize our relationships in ways that were more regenerative, more circular, more Indigenous, more feminine, more cooperative? So what are the values with which we organize our economic relationships? And how do we make a transition from forms of economic relationship that are based in violence, domination, and extraction to forms of economic relationship based in love, care, and community, or resilience, regeneration, interdependence?

So it's about understanding the history of the place you call home and figuring out what your responsibilities to that place are. And who are the caretakers of that place. Those who know the way care for the place and the people in it, and they show others how to care for the place, to care for the land, and to care for the people. So it's about being in right relationship with the stewards and caretakers of the place that you're in, helping to find ways to contribute to the thriving of that place and the people in it. And, you know, it's just as simple as that. And as challenging as that.

ROSHI NORMA: *The collective does not exist unless a critical mass of individuals come into a mutual relationship with each other. Spores in the environment come together, find themselves with each other, and then become something else. It only takes three people to form a critical mass towards a particular endeavor, if you're in mutuality with each other—which is different than whether you are in ideological agreement. When you have the conversations around values and shared destinations and those types of things, you're still in the realm of concept. When you're in mutuality, you have a felt sense of yourself and the other being. Sometimes when you're in crisis situations, it's actually people who are unable to communicate verbally with each other who are able to move with each other with more purpose than people who have to enter into a conversation about it. So the hopefulness of accelerated trauma, such as in a worldwide pandemic, is to interrupt the pattern of our reliance on needing to come within some kind of a structured way in which we think of change or transformation.*

KERRI: *It feels like we are situated in a messy and uncertain transition between where we are coming from and where we are going. How do we navigate this transition?*

Taj: *As the systems that we are in collapse, and we work to create space for new systems to emerge—based on a different set of values that honor life, honor our interdependence, honor the ways in which we need to care for each other in order for all of us to thrive—our job is to first recognize that there's no escape. That we are all inextricably embedded in the collapsing systems and the emerging systems. The question is, How skillfully can we draw energy out of the old collapsing systems and infuse that energy into the emerging systems? It's an energetic question, it's a spiritual question, and it's a material question. What I have found to be fruitful is that the more time I spend with others coming together to build what we need, the less harm and suffering we will experience in the transition and the collapse of the old systems and the emergence of the new systems.*

Teo: *I think about this on a very personal level as someone who has experienced gender transition. Prior to transition, I knew I was in crisis. I knew that where I was currently residing was not the whole of me. Living in that place was unsustainable, but I did not actually know the destination. I had hopes, I had visions, I knew other people's experiences, but I had no way to be certain that if I took that leap I would land somewhere I wanted to be. What I had was faith, what I had was community, what I had was the ability and the choice to use my pain to motivate me to change. That stuff fueled me to take a leap of faith but to do so with wise information. To begin to move forward on a path—and along the way continue to evaluate whether this path was bringing me closer to wholeness and calling me home. And I did that in relationship, I did that in community, I did that with other folks who were maybe slightly ahead of me in some ways; I certainly couldn't do it alone. The ability to hold where I might be heading had to be a collective effort. But ultimately it had to be about faith. Faith in my own birthright. Faith that I could move beyond the lie I'd been told.*

And I think about that in terms of this collective transition, because particularly in a white supremacist culture there is such a need for certainty, a need for perfection, a need to plan and know and guarantee. I don't think we can; I think it's inherently impossible to know exactly where we are going to end up. What I know and trust is that we individually and collectively have what we need in order to begin to move toward what can be. In us and in generations to come, we can nurture the tools that we need going forward. We can start something without having the exact answers, because we can trust one another to build as we go.

As a woodworker and artisan, there are two ways that I've seen people approach building. One way is that they plan to the T, every single step—and that's great when it works, but if one little thing doesn't go as planned, often things fall apart. The other way is through intuition, paired with some skill, where they feel into the process of making something. This second way is outside the dominant culture's comfort zone, but there are lots of us who come from cultures where leaning into something and intuitively building as we go is the way that it's always been. The need to know—and vet—the destination before beginning feels rooted in the small self, in ego, as opposed to asking, "Are we and am I worth the effort of trying?" We need to lay a groundwork of faith in one another and collective responsibility that we don't need to design an end product, we just need to begin where we are with what we have and trust that what we need next will come as we're doing the work.

ANASA: *We are working to cultivate a culture that is grounded in the core value of love. This is the gravitational center that brings us back to understanding the sacred nature of life and how to lovingly interact with ourselves, each other, and the planet in very practical ways that include practice and policy. If you want to behave lovingly to young people, start with changing the way we fund public schools, so that all children get the same level of service and support and are studying curricula that honor their intellectual and emotional intelligence, tell the truth, and prepare them to create and lead us into the future instead of only training them to be the workers. This act alone would advance the cause of wellness by leaps and bounds! In a culture of love, we begin with understanding what it means to love and nurture ourselves, and then we make sure that everyone else has access to those things. Love for self and love for the collective must exist at the same time, or true wellness is not possible.*

The transition is the difficult part, but we get through it by embodying the value of love from the beginning. Love with yourself including patience, belief, surrounding yourself with community and accountability. Love with others . . . How do you get through a hard conversation or a difficult time in a healthy way with someone that you love? You listen, you tell the truth, you learn to trust, be vulnerable, assume good intent, you hold others accountable to your agreements, and you set boundaries accordingly.

TAJ: *As our Movement Generation and Climate Justice Alliance friends remind us, the transition is inevitable. These systems are going to collapse. The only question is, Will the transition be just? Can we minimize the needless suffering that is inevitably going to come along with this transition? And that's where folks thinking about this through the lens of climate change remind us that every little bit that we do to accelerate this transition into new systems that honor life will save countless lives and reduce immeasurable suffering. Things are, and are going to be, brutally painful. Some people are continuing to just ask how they can make sure that they personally experience the least amount of that pain and divert that pain onto others—which is the basic thinking that created the whole crisis in the first place. And other people are asking ourselves how we can come together in a way that we thrive through the transition. Not just survive the transition, but thrive through the transition. How we can party our way to a better, more sustainable world by making sure that everybody gets what they need through the transition?*

What's important about that is, through our dance, and our song, and our celebration, and our mourning, and our grief, what we will communicate is that we are not afraid. To the last breath, we are not afraid. Because we know who we are, and we know we are a continuation of those who came before us, and we know those who come after us will be a continuation of us, and there is nothing to fear. We were never born and we will never die. Nothing to fear.

EPILOGUE

This book-writing process taught me a lot about emergence. The definition of emergence is "the process of coming into view or becoming exposed after being concealed."[1] It is to bring into the light. And while being a truth-teller was my intention when I set out to write this book, I could never have imagined the unraveling and unveiling that would follow. How the truth would demand everything from me—the death of who I thought I was before writing this book and the birth of the me that I am yet to fully understand and embody.

The language of emergence is listening, allowing oneself to always be moved and changed, tuning in to the wisdom that is beyond words and language. And remembering—always remembering that we are not the first and we will not be the last. There will always be those who came before us and those who are yet to come. Time is not linear, which means we are the past, present, and future. We are the ancestors and we are descendants. We are the teachers and we are the students. We are the end of one thing and the beginning of another.

And in the spirit of nonclosure, this journey (as with most processes of transformation) has left me with more questions than answers. And much more conviction and commitment for the future I believe is possible.

I am on a forever mission to understand more clearly who I am beyond what whiteness, individualism, and capitalism have told and taught me I am. The answer calls me back to retrieve the parts of me that have been forgotten and lost to the project of white, Christian, capitalist supremacy. To get in relationship with the medicine of my Celtic ancestors who understood the intimate and interdependent relationship of "as above, so below, as within so without" (as depicted in the Tree of Life, which is at the heart of Celtic culture). Its wisdom invites us to confront and challenge whatever goes against nature and do whatever is necessary to bring our world into harmony and balance.

What I know now, at the end of this journey and the beginning of the next, is that there's more—more to learn, more to do, more to dream, more to love.

Just *more*.

KEEP GOING: A RESOURCE LIST

I hope this book will inspire you to learn more, dig deeper, and follow the people who know the way. Here's a list of books, podcasts, and organizations that have inspired and informed my path.

Decolonize (chapter 1)

BOOKS

Decolonizing Wealth: Indigenous Wisdom to Heal Divides and Restore Balance, Edgar Villanueva

Sacred Instructions: Indigenous Wisdom for Living Spirit-Based Change, Sherri Mitchell (Weh'na Ha'mu Kwasset)

Braiding Sweetgrass: Indigenous Wisdom, Scientific Knowledge, and Teachings of Plants, Robin Wall Kimmerer

To Be a Water Protector: The Rise of the Wiindigoo Slayers, Winona LaDuke

There There, Tommy Orange

Carry: A Memoir of Survival on Stolen Land, Toni Jensen

In Times of Terror, Wage Beauty, Mark Gonzales

PODCASTS

Let's Talk Native with John Kane

Coffee with My Ma, Kaniehti:io Horn

Decolonizing Fitness, Ilya Parker and Candace Liger

All My Relations, Matika Wilbur, Adrienne Keene, and Desi Small-Rodriguez

Telling Our Twisted Histories, Kaniehti:io Horn

ORGANIZATIONS

Sogorea Te' Land Trust: https://sogoreate-landtrust.org/

Seeding Sovereignty: https://seedingsovereignty.org/

Climate Justice Alliance: https://climatejusticealliance.org/

Indigenous Climate Action: https://indigenousclimateaction.com/

NDN Collective: https://ndncollective.org/

Decolonizing Wealth Project: https://decolonizingwealth.com/

Healing Justice (chapter 2)

BOOKS

Politics of Trauma: Somatics, Healing, and Social Justice, Staci Haines

Peace from Anxiety: Get Grounded, Build Resilience and Stay Connected Amidst the Chaos, Hala Khouri

The Body Keeps the Score: Mind, Brain and Body in the Transformation of Trauma, Bessel van der Kolk

Restorative Yoga for Ethnic and Race-Based Stress and Trauma, Gail Parker

Brilliant Imperfection: Grappling with Cure, Eli Clare

Care Work: Dreaming Disability Justice, Leah Lakshmi Piepzna-Samarasinha

A Disability History of the United States, Kim E. Nielsen

All the Weight of Our Dreams: On Living Racialized Autism, edited by Lydia X. Z. Brown, E. Ashkenazy, and Morénike Giwa Onaiwu

Spectrums: Autistic Transgender People in Their Own Words, edited by Maxfield Sparrow

PODCASTS

Fortification Podcast: Spiritual Sustenance for Movement, Caitlin Breedlove

La Cura, Mijente Support Committee

Finding Our Way, Prentis Hemphill

Emergent Strategy, Sage Crump, Mia Herndon, and adrienne maree brown

ORGANIZATIONS

Sins Invalid: https://sinsinvalid.org/

Project LETS: https://projectlets.org/

Disability Visibility Project: https://disabilityvisibilityproject.com/

Autistic Self Advocacy Network: https://autisticadvocacy.org/

ADAPT: https://adapt.org/

Healing Histories Project: https://healinghistoriesproject.com/

The Embodiment Institute: https://theembodimentinstitute.org/

Kindred Southern Healing Justice Collective: http://kindredsouthern hjcollective.org/

Wellness Equity (chapter 3)

BOOKS

Inflamed: Deep Medicine and the Anatomy of Injustice, Rupa Marya and Raj Patel

The Health Gap: The Challenge of an Unequal World, Michael Marmot

The Wellness Syndrome, Carl Cederström and André Spicer

Natural Causes: An Epidemic of Wellness, the Certainty of Dying, and Killing Ourselves to Live Longer, Barbara Ehrenreich

Skill in Action: Radicalizing Your Yoga Practice to Create a Just World, Michelle Cassandra Johnson

Embrace Yoga's Roots: Courageous Ways to Deepen Your Yoga Practice, Susanna Barkataki

Against Purity: Living Ethically in Compromised Times, Alexis Shotwell

Revolution of the Soul: Awaken to Love through Raw Truth, Radical Healing, and Conscious Action, Seane Corn

PODCASTS

Good Ancestor Podcast, Layla Saad

Black Girl in Om, Lauren Ash

Matriarch Movement, Shayla Oulette Stonechild

Yoga Is Dead, Tejal Patel and Jesal Parikh

You Good Sis?, The Slaters

CTZN, CTZNWELL

ORGANIZATIONS

BEAM (Black Emotional and Mental Health Collective): https://beam.community/

Black Girl in Om: https://blackgirlinom.com/

Indigenous Circle of Wellness: https://icowellness.com/

Latinx Therapists Action Network: https://latinxtherapistsactionnetwork.org/

The Loveland Foundation: https://thelovelandfoundation.org/

Reclamation Ventures: https://reclamationventures.co/

Black Yoga Teachers Alliance: https://blackyogateachersalliance.org/

Amplify and Activate: https://amplifyandactivate.com/

Off the Mat, Into the World: https://offthematintotheworld.org/

Transforming Hearts Collective: http://transformingheartscollective.org/

The Wellness of We: https://thewellnessofwe.com/

CTZNWELL: https://ctznwell.org/

Collective Care (chapter 4)

BOOKS

The Body Is Not an Apology: The Power of Radical Self-Love, Sonya Renee Taylor

Belly of the Beast: The Politics of Anti-Fatness as Anti-Blackness, Da'Shaun L. Harrison

Body Respect: What Conventional Health Books Get Wrong, Leave Out, and Just Plain Fail to Understand about Weight, Linda Bacon and Lucy Aphramor

You Are Your Best Thing: Vulnerability, Shame Resilience, and the Black Experience, Tarana Burke

How to Do Nothing: Resisting the Attention Economy, Jenny Odell

Work Won't Love You Back: How Devotion to Our Jobs Keeps Us Exploited, Exhausted, and Alone, Sarah Jaffe

The Real Wealth of Nations: Creating a Caring Economics, Riane Eisler

The New Better Off: Reinventing the American Dream, Courtney E. Martin

Mutualism: Building the Next Economy from the Ground Up, Sara Horowitz

Mutual Aid: Building Solidarity during This Crisis (and the Next), Dean Spade

PODCASTS

She's All Fat, Sophia Carter-Kahn

Maintenance Phase, Michael Hobbes and Aubrey Gordon

How to Survive the End of the World, Autumn Brown and adrienne maree brown

Stories from Home: Living the Just Transition, Climate Justice Alliance

Did We Go Too Far?, Tré Vasquez and Layel Camargo

ORGANIZATIONS

Movement Generation Justice and Ecology Project: https://movement
generation.org/

HEAL Food Alliance: https://healfoodalliance.org/

New Economy Coalition: https://neweconomy.net/

Center for Partnership Systems: https://centerforpartnership.org/

The Nap Ministry: https://thenapministry.wordpress.com/

From Me to We (chapter 5)

BOOKS

How We Show Up: Reclaiming Family, Friendship, and Community, Mia
Birdsong

Holding Change: The Way of Emergent Strategy Facilitation and Mediation,
adrienne maree brown

The Art of Gathering: How We Meet and Why It Matters, Priya Parker

Radical Belonging: How to Survive and Thrive in an Unjust World, Lindo
Bacon

Community: The Structure of Belonging, Peter Block

Bowling Alone: The Collapse and Revival of American Community, Robert
D. Putnam

Big Friendship: How We Keep Each Other Close, Aminatou Sow and Ann
Friedman

PODCASTS

Solidarity Is This, Deepa Iyer

We Rise, We Rise Production

Hear to Slay, Roxane Gay and Tressie McMillan Cottom

On Being, Krista Tippett

ORGANIZATIONS

The BIG We: https://thebigwe.com/

Movement Strategy Center: https://movementstrategy.org/

Othering and Belonging Institute: https://belonging.berkeley.edu/

Resonance Network: https://resonance-network.org/

Thrive Network: https://thrivenetwork.org/

Wellness beyond Whiteness (chapter 6)

BOOKS

Me and White Supremacy: How to Recognise Your Privilege, Combat Racism and Change the World, Layla F. Saad

Radical Dharma: Talking Race, Love, and Liberation, Rev. angel Kyodo williams, Lama Rod Owens, and Jasmine Syedullah

My Grandmother's Hands: Racialized Trauma and the Pathway to Mending Our Hearts and Bodies, Resmaa Menakem

The Racial Healing Handbook: Practical Activities to Help You Challenge Privilege, Confront Systemic Racism, and Engage in Collective Healing, Anneliese A. Singh

Hood Feminism: Notes from the Women That a Movement Forgot, Mikki Kendall

Caste: The Origins of Our Discontents, Isabel Wilkerson

Stamped from the Beginning: The Definitive History of Racist Ideas in America, Ibram X. Kendi

The New Jim Crow: Mass Incarceration in the Age of Colorblindness, Michelle Alexander

Minor Feelings: An Asian American Reckoning, Cathy Park Hong

Fumbling towards Repair: A Workbook for Community Accountability Facilitators, Mariame Kaba and Shira Hassan

Change Everything: Racial Capitalism and the Case for Abolition, Ruth Wilson Gilmore

Becoming Abolitionists: Police, Protests, and the Pursuit of Freedom, Derecka Purnell

We Do This 'Til We Free Us: Abolitionist Organizing and Transforming Justice, Mariame Kaba

Winners Take All: The Elite Charade of Changing the World, Anand Giridharadas

PODCASTS

Beyond Prisons, Kim Wilson and Brian Nam-Sonenstein

1619, Nikole Hannah-Jones (*New York Times*)

The Work, Nicole Cardoza (Anti-Racism Daily)

Scene on Radio, "Seeing White," John Biewen and Chenjerai Kumanyika

Abolition Is for Everybody, Taina Angeli Vargas, Lee Gibson, and Ra Jaini

ORGANIZATIONS

The Movement for Black Lives: https://m4bl.org/

Black Youth Project 100: https://byp100.org/

Transform Harm: https://transformharm.org/

Just Practice: https://just-practice.org/

Bay Area Transformative Justice Collective: https://batjc.wordpress.com/

Project Nia: https://project-nia.org/

Abolitionist Futures: https://abolitionistfutures.com/

The Politics of Belonging (chapter 7)

BOOKS

Dear America: Notes of an Undocumented Citizen, Jose Antonio Vargas

Borderlands / La Frontera: The New Mestiza, Gloria Anzaldúa

Sanctuary, Paola Mendoza and Abby Sher

The Purpose of Power: How We Come Together When We Fall Apart, Alicia Garza

The Sum of Us: What Racism Costs Everyone and How We Can Prosper Together, Heather McGhee

Defund Fear: Safety without Police, Prisons, and Punishment, Zach Norris

We Will Not Cancel Us: And Other Dreams of Transformative Justice, adrienne maree brown

The Gardens of Democracy: A New American Story of Citizenship, the Economy, and the Role of Government, Eric Liu and Nick Hanauer

Beautiful Trouble: A Toolbox for Revolution, Andrew Boyd

See No Stranger: A Memoir and Manifesto of Revolutionary Love, Valarie Kaur

Healing Resistance: A Radically Different Response to Harm, Kazu Haga

Hope in the Dark: Untold Histories, Wild Possibilities, Rebecca Solnit

PODCASTS

How to Citizen with Baratunde, Baratunde Thurston

Words to Win By, Anat Shenker-Osorio

Who Belongs?, Othering and Belonging Institute

Pod Save America, Crooked Media

Betches Sup, Amanda Duberman

ORGANIZATIONS

Working Families Party: https://workingfamilies.org/

Mijente: https://mijente.net/

Southerners on New Ground: https://southernersonnewground.org/

Justice Democrats: https://justicedemocrats.com/

Women's March: https://womensmarch.com/

GRATITUDE

I spent many weeks reckoning with acknowledgments. How does one begin to recognize and appreciate the many origins of one's learning and evolution? Who I have become is because of you—all of you who have loved me and challenged me to show up for the assignment I've been given. These pages are a culmination of your care, guidance, and support along the way.

Thank you to the most amazing literary team who stuck with me through this long journey and said "I believe in you" when I needed to hear it most. Alex Kapitan (https://radicalcopyeditor.com/), Linda Sparrowe, Teo Drake, Tim McKee, Shayna Keyles, Laura Sharkey, and the entire North Atlantic Books family. And to Gareth Esersky from Carole Mann Agency who took the leap with me.

Thank you to the long lineage of teachers who have inspired me with not just your wisdom but your example. I am changed because of you. Taj James, Ruby Sales, Rev. angel Kyodo williams, adrienne maree brown, Marianne Manilov, Seane Corn, Dr. Jasmine Syedullah, Mark Gonzales, Gina Breedlove, Lama Rod Owens, Anasa Troutman, Tracee Stanley, and Roshi Norma Wong.

Thank you to the fierce witches and warlocks in my life who I can always rely on to speak unapologetic truth and hold me to the fire. Michelle, Melody, Seane, Nikki, Heidi, Carinne, Terri, Carrington, Suzanne, Hala, Anita, Micky, Leigh, Janet, Shannon and Ryan.

Thank you to my family, who loves me despite everything. Mom, Caitlin, Brian, Larissa, Kaia, Jo Bo, Dad, Carole, Steven, Scott.

Thank you, Trevor, for witnessing me in my most brutal and beautiful moments. Thank you for pushing me to write with my whole heart. Thank you for reminding me not to be scared. Thank you for sourdough bread. Thank you for music.

And thank you, ancestors who I carry with me always. Joe, Muffy, Ruth, Renee, Emily, Eva.

NOTES

Introduction

1 "2018 Global Wellness Economy Monitor," Global Wellness Institute, July 15, 2021, https://globalwellnessinstitute.org/industry-research/2018 -global-wellness-economy-monitor/.

2 Jack Ewing, "United States Is the Richest Country in the World, and It Has the Biggest Wealth Gap," *New York Times*, September 23, 2020, www .nytimes.com/2020/09/23/business/united-states-is-the-richest-country -in-the-world-and-it-has-the-biggest-wealth-gap.html.

3 Kelly Kerri, "The Privilege of Well-Being," video, TEDx Talks, May 27, 2016, www.youtube.com/watch?v=CZowld1g7Qo.

4 Bobbie Harro, "The Cycle of Liberation," in *Readings for Diversity and Social Justice: An Anthology on Racism, Antisemitism, Sexism, Heterosexism, Ableism, and Classism*, ed. Maurianne Adams et al. (New York: Routledge, 2000), 463.

Chapter 1

1 Hannah Hartig and Carroll Doherty, "Two Decades Later, the Enduring Legacy of 9/11," Pew Research Center, September 2, 2021, www.pewresearch .org/politics/2021/09/02/two-decades-later-the-enduring-legacy-of-9-11 /#the-new-normal-the-threat-of-terrorism-after-9-11.

2 Michele Gelfand, "After 9/11, Americans United. Today, Fake Threats Divide Us," *Time*, September 11, 2018, https://time.com/5392451 /september-11-tightness-immigration-fears/.

3 Naomi Klein, *The Shock Doctrine: The Rise of Disaster Capitalism* (New York: Picador, 2008).

4   "Dutch Colonization," US National Park Service, accessed September 13, 2021, https://www.nps.gov/nr/travel/kingston/colonization.htm; "Henry Hudson Entering New York Bay, September 11, 1609, from a Painting by Edward Moran," New York State Archives (New York State Education Department), accessed September 5, 2021, www.archives.nysed.gov/education/henry-hudson-entering-new-york-bay-september-11-1609-painting.

5   "The True, Dark History of Thanksgiving," Citizen Potawatomi Nation, November 25, 2020, www.potawatomi.org/blog/2020/11/25/the-true-dark-history-of-thanksgiving/.

6   Lauren Kent, "European Colonizers Killed So Many Native Americans That It Changed the Global Climate, Researchers Say," CNN, February 2, 2019, www.cnn.com/2019/02/01/world/european-colonization-climate-change-trnd/index.html.

7   Ruth Hopkins, "Of Scalps and Savages: How Colonial Language Enforces Discrimination against Indigenous Peoples," Last Real Indians, March 31, 2013, https://lastrealindians.com/videos/2013/3/31/of-scalps-and-savages-how-colonial-language-enforces-discrimination-against-indigenous-peoples-by-ruth-hopkins.

8   Lindsay Koshgarian, Ashik Siddique, and Lorah Steichen, "State of Insecurity: The Cost of Militarization Since 9/11," Institute for Policy Studies, August 2021, https://ips-dc.org/wp-content/uploads/2021/08/State-of-Insecurity-The-Cost-of-Militarization-Since-911.pdf.

9   Edgar Villanueva, *Decolonizing Wealth: Indigenous Wisdom to Heal Divides and Restore Balance* (Oakland, CA: Berrett-Koehler, 2021).

10 Susanna Barkataki, *Embrace Yoga's Roots: Courageous Ways to Deepen Your Yoga Practice* (Orlando, FL: Ignite Yoga and Wellness Institute, 2020), 48.

11 "House Session," video, C-SPAN, October 17, 2001, www.c-span.org/video/?166723-1%2Fhouse-session.

12 Valarie Kaur, "A Sikh Prayer for America on November 9th, 2016," November 11, 2016, https://valariekaur.com/2016/11/a-sikh-prayer-for-america-on-november-9th-2016/.

13 Pema Chödrön, *When Things Fall Apart: Heart Advice for Difficult Times*, 20th anniv. ed. (Boston: Shambhala, 2016), 14.

14 Cynthia Occelli, home page, accessed September 30, 2021, www.cynthiaoccelli.com.

15 *Merriam-Webster Dictionary*, s.v. "dismembering," accessed October 11, 2021, www.merriam-webster.com/dictionary/dismembering.

16 Taj James, in discussion with the author, August 1, 2021.

17 Sherri Mitchell, *Sacred Instructions: Indigenous Wisdom for Living Spirit-Based Change* (Berkeley, CA: North Atlantic Books, 2018), 40.

18 Michelle Schenandoah et al., "Rematriation: Returning the Sacred to the Mother," *Rematriation*, May 13, 2021, https://rematriation.com/.

19 Mitchell, *Sacred Instructions*, 55.

20 Malkia Devich-Cyril, "Grief Belongs in Social Movements. Can We Embrace It?," *In These Times,* July 28, 2021, https://inthesetimes.com /article/freedom-grief-healing-death-liberation-movements.

21 Kanyon CoyoteWoman Sayers-Roods, "EmergingSF Honors Native Land," Kanyon Konsulting LLC, June 11, 2018, https://kanyonkonsulting .com/emergingsf-honors-native-land/.

22 "Return Land / Land Return," Sogorea Te' Land Trust, July 20, 2021, https://sogoreate-landtrust.org/return-land/.

23 Qwul'sih'yah'maht et al., "Homework: Questions about 'Home,'" Catalyst Project, accessed October 24, 2021, https://collectiveliberation.org /wp-content/uploads/2018/10/Indigenous-Resistance-Homework.pdf.

Chapter 2

1 "Chronic Diseases in America," Centers for Disease Control and Prevention, January 12, 2021, www.cdc.gov/chronicdisease/resources/info graphic/chronic-diseases.htm; "Health and Economic Costs of Chronic Diseases," National Center for Chronic Disease Prevention and Health Promotion (Centers for Disease Control and Prevention), June 23, 2021, www.cdc.gov/chronicdisease/about/costs/index.htm; Rabah Kamal and Julie Hudman, "What Do We Know about Spending Related to Public Health in the U.S. and Comparable Countries?," Peterson-KFF Health System Tracker, September 30, 2020, www.healthsystemtracker.org /chart-collection/what-do-we-know-about-spending-related-to-public -health-in-the-u-s-and-comparable-countries/.

2 "National Health Expenditure Data," US Centers for Medicare and Medicaid Services, 2019, www.cms.gov/Research-Statistics-Data-and -Systems/Statistics-Trends-and-Reports/NationalHealthExpendData /NationalHealthAccountsHistorical; "France GDP," Trading Economics, accessed September 12, 2021, https://tradingeconomics.com/france /gdp; Karen Feldscher, "What's Behind High U.S. Health Care Costs,"

Harvard Gazette, March 13, 2018, https://news.harvard.edu/gazette
/story/2018/03/u-s-pays-more-for-health-care-with-worse-population
-health-outcomes/.

3 Wendell Berry, *The Gift of Good Land: Further Essays Cultural and Agricultural* (Berkeley, CA: Counterpoint, 2009), xiii.

4 Lynn Payer, *Disease-Mongers: How Doctors, Drug Companies, and Insurers Are Making You Feel Sick* (New York: Wiley, 1992).

5 Laura Clark, "How Halitosis Became a Medical Condition with a 'Cure,'" *Smithsonian*, January 29, 2015, www.smithsonianmag.com/smart-news
/marketing-campaign-invented-halitosis-180954082/.

6 Rebecca Farley, "Do Pharmaceutical Companies Spend More on Marketing than Research and Development?," PharmacyChecker, April 21, 2021, www.pharmacychecker.com/askpc/pharma-marketing-research
-development/; Karl Evers-Hillstrom, "Big Pharma Continues to Top Lobbying Spending," OpenSecrets, October 25, 2019, www.opensecrets
.org/news/2019/10/big-pharma-continues-to-top-lobbying-spending/; Julia Belluz, "Doctors and Hospitals Got at Least $3.5 Billion from Industry in Just Five Months," Vox, September 30, 2014, www.vox.com
/2014/9/30/6868897/you-can-now-search-for-your-doctors-pharma
-payments-online-sunshine-act.

7 "Understanding the Epidemic," Centers for Disease Control and Prevention, March 17, 2021, www.cdc.gov/opioids/basics/epidemic.html.

8 Donovan Keene, "Big Pharma: The International Reach of the Opioid Crisis," *Harvard Political Review*, May 4, 2020, https://harvardpolitics
.com/big-pharma/.

9 Alex Kacik, "Few Women Reach Healthcare Leadership Roles," Modern Healthcare, May 22, 2019, www.modernhealthcare.com/operations
/few-women-reach-healthcare-leadership-roles.

10 Barbara Ehrenreich and Deirdre English, *Witches, Midwives and Nurses: A History of Women Healers*, 2nd ed. (New York: Feminist Press at the City University of New York, 2010), 28.

11 Jonathan Mooney, "How, Exactly, Did We Come Up with What Counts as 'Normal'?," Literary Hub, August 16, 2019, https://lithub.com/how
-exactly-did-we-come-up-with-what-counts-as-normal/.

12 Jessica Helfand, "Darwin, Expression and the Lasting Legacy of Eugenics," *Scientific American*, August 13, 2020, www.scientificamerican.com
/article/darwin-expression-and-the-lasting-legacy-of-eugenics/.

13 "How Samuel Morton Got It Wrong," Learning for Justice (Southern Poverty Law Center), May 13, 2015, www.learningforjustice.org /magazine/how-samuel-morton-got-it-wrong.

14 Brendan Wolfe, "Buck v. Bell (1927)," Encyclopedia Virginia (Virginia Humanities), accessed September 5, 2021, https://encyclopediavirginia .org/entries/buck-v-bell-1927/.

15 Cris Haest, "The History of Forced Sterilization," Saenz-Rodriguez and Associates, November 30, 2020, www.sralawonline.com/the-history-of -forced-sterilization.

16 Sonya Renee Taylor, *The Body Is Not an Apology: The Power of Radical Self-Love* (Oakland, CA: Berrett-Koehler, 2018), 36.

17 Taylor, *Not an Apology*, 72.

18 Mia Mingus, "Medical Industrial Complex Visual," Leaving Evidence, February 6, 2015, https://leavingevidence.wordpress.com/2015/02/06 /medical-industrial-complex-visual/.

19 Robert Crawford, "Healthism and the Medicalization of Everyday Life," *International Journal of Health Services* 10, no. 3 (1980): 365–88, https://doi .org/10.2190/3h2h-3xjn-3kay-g9ny.

20 Jonathan Metzl, "Introduction: Why 'Against Health'?," in *Against Health: How Health Became the New Morality*, ed. Jonathan Metzl and Anna Kirkland (New York: New York University Press, 2010), 1.

21 Assistant Secretary for Public Affairs, "Pre-Existing Conditions," US Department of Health and Human Services, January 31, 2017, www.hhs .gov/healthcare/about-the-aca/pre-existing-conditions/index.html.

22 Paula Braveman and Laura Gottlieb, "The Social Determinants of Health: It's Time to Consider the Causes of the Causes," *Public Health Reports* 129, no. S2 (2014): 19–31, https://doi.org/10.1177%2F00333549141291S206.

23 Dan Peters, "Pathologizing the Human Condition," The Health Care Blog, September 1, 2013, https://thehealthcareblog.com/blog/2013/09/01 /pathologizing-the-human-condition/.

24 Neel Burton, "When Homosexuality Stopped Being a Mental Disorder," *Psychology Today*, September 18, 2015, www.psychologytoday.com/us /blog/hide-and-seek/201509/when-homosexuality-stopped-being-mental -disorder; Srishti Uppal, "The Case for and Problems with the Inclusion of Gender Dysphoria in the DSM," Gaysi, December 24, 2020, https:// gaysifamily.com/2020/12/24/the-case-for-and-problems-with-the-inclusion -of-gender-dysphoria-in-the-dsm/.

25 Eli Clare, *Brilliant Imperfection: Grappling with Cure* (Durham, NC: Duke University Press, 2017), 14.

26 Leah Lakshmi Piepzna-Samarasinha, "Not over It, Not Fixed and Living a Life Worth Living: A Disability Justice View of Survivorhood," *Herizons*, accessed September 6, 2021, http://www.herizons.ca/node/725.

27 Leah Lakshmi Piepzna-Samarasinha, *Care Work: Dreaming Disability Justice* (Vancouver, BC: Arsenal Pulp, 2018), 103.

28 adrienne maree brown, *Emergent Strategy: Shaping Change, Changing Worlds* (Chico, CA: AK Press, 2017), 35.

29 Staci Haines, *The Politics of Trauma: Somatics, Healing, and Social Justice* (Berkeley, CA: North Atlantic Books, 2019), 74.

30 Peter A. Levine with Ann Frederick, *Waking the Tiger: Healing Trauma* (Berkeley, CA: North Atlantic Books, 1997), 34.

31 *The Wisdom of Trauma*, directed by Zaya Benazzo and Maurizio Benazzo (Science and Nonduality, 2021), https://thewisdomoftrauma.com/.

32 Piepzna-Samarasinha, *Care Work*, 102.

33 Mia Mingus, "Changing the Framework: Disability Justice," Leaving Evidence, February 12, 2011, https://leavingevidence.wordpress.com/2011/02/12/changing-the-framework-disability-justice/.

34 "Our History," Kindred Southern Healing Justice Collective, accessed September 12, 2021, http://kindredsouthernhjcollective.org/our-history/.

35 "Healing by Choice!," Allied Media Projects, August 24, 2021, https://alliedmedia.org/speaker-projects/healing-by-choice.

36 Cheryl Strayed, *Brave Enough* (New York: Knopf, 2015), 10.

Chapter 3

1 Daniela Blei, "The False Promises of Wellness Culture," JSTOR Daily, January 4, 2017, https://daily.jstor.org/the-false-promises-of-wellness-culture/.

2 Blei, "False Promises."

3 Philip Deslippe, "Yoga Landed in the U.S. Way Earlier Than You'd Think—and Fitness Was Not the Point," History.com, June 20, 2019, www.history.com/news/yoga-vivekananda-america.

4 Sonia Faleiro, "'The Goddess Pose,' by Michelle Goldberg," *New York Times*, July 13, 2015, www.nytimes.com/2015/07/19/books/review/the-goddess-pose-by-michelle-goldberg.html.

5 "The Immigration Act of 1924 (The Johnson-Reed Act)," Office of the Historian (US Department of State), accessed September 13, 2021, https:// history.state.gov/milestones/1921-1936/immigration-act.

6 "2018 Global Wellness Economy Monitor," Global Wellness Institute, July 15, 2021, https://globalwellnessinstitute.org/industry-research/2018 -global-wellness-economy-monitor/.

7 "2018 Global Wellness Economy Monitor."

8 "FastStats: Leading Causes of Death," National Center for Health Statistics (Centers for Disease Control and Prevention), March 1, 2021, www .cdc.gov/nchs/fastats/leading-causes-of-death.htm.

9 Rachel Charlene Lewis, "Netflix's 'The Goop Lab' Turns Fear and Trauma into Profit," Bitch Media, January 24, 2020, www.bitchmedia.org/article /netflix-the-goop-lab-Gwyneth-Paltrow-review.

10 Wullianallur Raghupathi and Viju Raghupathi, "An Empirical Study of Chronic Diseases in the United States: A Visual Analytics Approach to Public Health," *International Journal of Environmental Research and Public Health* 15, no. 3 (March 2018): 431, https://dx.doi.org/10.3390%2Fi jerph15030431; Gabriela R. Oates et al., "Sociodemographic Patterns of Chronic Disease," *American Journal of Preventive Medicine* 52, no. S1 (January 2017): S31–S39, https://dx.doi.org/10.1016%2Fj.amepre.2016.09.004; "Racial and Ethnic Disparities Continue in Pregnancy-Related Deaths," Centers for Disease Control and Prevention, September 6, 2019, https:// www.cdc.gov/media/releases/2019/p0905-racial-ethnic-disparities -pregnancy-deaths.html; Mark DeCambre, "The Richest 10% of Households Now Represent 70% of All U.S. Wealth," MarketWatch, May 31, 2019, https://www.marketwatch.com/story/the-richest-10-of -households-now-represent-70-of-all-us-wealth-2019-05-24; Josh Rovner and Keeda Haynes, "Black Disparities in Youth Incarceration," Sentencing Project, July 15, 2021, www.sentencingproject.org/publications/black -disparities-youth-incarceration/.

11 "Life Expectancy vs. Income in the United States," Health Inequality Project, accessed September 13, 2021, https://healthinequality.org/.

12 Chabeli Carrazana, "Barriers for Black Women Set U.S. Economy Back by $500 Billion, Report Finds," The 19th, June 8, 2021, https://19thnews .org/2021/06/black-women-wage-gap/.

13 Carl Cederström and André Spicer, *The Wellness Syndrome* (Cambridge, UK: Polity, 2015), 133.

14 Cederström and Spicer, *Wellness Syndrome.*

15 Laurie Penny, "Life-Hacks of the Poor and Aimless," *Baffler*, July 8, 2016, https://thebaffler.com/latest/laurie-penny-self-care.

16 Raghupathi and Raghupathi, "Chronic Diseases in the United States."

17 Chloe Ann-King, "'Positive Attitude' Bullshit: On the Dangers of 'Radical Self-Love,'" July 8, 2015, https://millennialposse.wordpress.com/2015/07/08/positive-attitude-bullshit-on-the-dangers-of-radical-self-love-2/.

18 Gopal K. Singh et al., "Social Determinants of Health in the United States: Addressing Major Health Inequality Trends for the Nation, 1935–2016," *International Journal of Maternal and Child Health and AIDS* 6, no. 2 (2017): 139–64, https://dx.doi.org/10.21106%2Fijma.236.

19 Roge Karma, "The Gross Inequality of Death in America," *New Republic*, May 10, 2019, https://newrepublic.com/article/153870/inequality-death-america-life-expectancy-gap.

20 Sabrina Tavernise and Albert Sun, "Same City, but Very Different Life Spans," *New York Times*, April 28, 2015, www.nytimes.com/interactive/2015/04/29/health/life-expectancy-nyc-chi-atl-richmond.html#nyc.

21 Yasmeen Khan, "Poverty and Hardship Make Life Shorter in Brownsville," WNYC, May 28, 2017, www.wnyc.org/story/poverty-and-hardships-make-life-shorter-brownsville/.

22 "Infant Mortality and African Americans," Office of Minority Health (US Department of Health and Human Services), accessed September 13, 2021, https://minorityhealth.hhs.gov/omh/browse.aspx?lvl=4&lvlid=23; Jamila Taylor et al., "Eliminating Racial Disparities in Maternal and Infant Mortality," Center for American Progress, May 2, 2019, www.americanprogress.org/issues/women/reports/2019/05/02/469186/eliminating-racial-disparities-maternal-infant-mortality/.

23 "Racial and Ethnic Disparities Continue in Pregnancy-Related Deaths," Centers for Disease Control and Prevention, September 6, 2019, www.cdc.gov/media/releases/2019/p0905-racial-ethnic-disparities-pregnancy-deaths.html.

24 Leslie Farrington, "How the CDC and Others Are Failing Black Women during Childbirth," STAT, September 18, 2020, www.statnews.com/2020/09/18/how-the-cdc-and-others-are-failing-black-women-during-childbirth/.

25 Taylor et al., "Eliminating Racial Disparities."

26 Paul Farmer, *Pathologies of Power: Health, Human Rights, and the New War on the Poor* (Berkeley: University of California Press, 2003), 6.

27 Gina Crosley-Corcoran, "Explaining White Privilege to a Broke White Person," Equality Includes You, October 10, 2019, https://medium.com /equality-includes-you/explaining-white-privilege-to-a-broke-white -person-2239d9d2470b.

28 Kriston McIntosh, Emily Moss, Ryan Nunn, and Jay Shambaugh, "Examining the Black-White Wealth Gap," Brookings, February 27, 2020, www.brookings.edu/blog/up-front/2020/02/27/examining-the -black-white-wealth-gap/.

29 Jennifer Cheeseman and Danielle Taylor, "Do People with Disabilities Earn Equal Pay?," US Census Bureau, March 21, 2019, www.census .gov/library/stories/2019/03/do-people-with-disabilities-earn-equal -pay.html.

30 Mitch Kellaway, "Report: Trans Americans Four Times More Likely to Live in Poverty," *Advocate*, February 18, 2015, www.advocate.com/politics /transgender/2015/02/18/report-trans-americans-four-times-more-likely -live-poverty.

31 "Use It and Lose It: The Outsize Effect of U.S. Consumption on the Environment," *Scientific American*, September 14, 2012, www.scientificamerican .com/article/american-consumption-habits/.

32 Ruby Sales, "Good Medicine: Decolonizing Our Memory," video, Facebook, May 12, 2021, https://fb.watch/8NiwcILBFe/.

Chapter 4

1 Brené Brown, *The Gifts of Imperfection: Let Go of Who You Think You're Supposed to Be and Embrace Who You Are* (Center City, MN: Hazelden, 2010), 57.

2 Anne Lamott, *Bird by Bird: Some Instruction on Writing and Life* (New York: Anchor Books, 2019), 27.

3 "Nikki Myers: On Overcoming Addiction through Yoga and the 12-Steps," interview by Julia Hanlon, *Running on Om* podcast, episode 191, March 2014, https://runningonom.com/podcast-191/.

4 Melody Moore, in discussion with the author, August 5, 2018.

5 Sabrina Strings, *Fearing the Black Body: The Racial Origins of Fat Phobia* (New York: New York University Press, 2019), 211.

6 Da'Shaun L. Harrison, *Belly of the Beast: The Politics of Anti-Fatness as Anti-Blackness* (Berkeley, CA: North Atlantic Books, 2021), 37.

7   "Attempts to Lose Weight Among Adults in the United States, 2013–2016,"
    Centers for Disease Control and Prevention, NCHS Data Brief No. 313,
    July 12, 2018, www.cdc.gov/nchs/products/databriefs/db313.htm.

8   Rebecca Stamp, "Average Person Will Try 126 Fad Diets in Their Life-
    time, Poll Claims," *Independent*, January 8, 2020, www.independent.co
    .uk/life-style/diet-weight-loss-food-unhealthy-eating-habits-a9274676.html.

9   "The Number-One Reason Kids Are Bullied," Yahoo, July 8, 2015,
    https://www.yahoo.com/lifestyle/the-number-one-reason-kids-are
    -bullied-123555176933.html; C. Conover, "Too Fat to Be a Princess? Study
    Shows Young Girls Worry about Body Image," UCF Today, November
    26, 2009, www.ucf.edu/news/too-fat-to-be-a-princess-study-shows-young
    -girls-worry-about-body-image/.

10 Virginia Sole-Smith, "Meet the Thin White Men Who Rebranded Diet-
    ing as 'Wellness,'" *Bitch*, February 4, 2019, www.bitchmedia.org/article
    /well-actually-wellness/thin-white-men-and-rebranding-diet-culture/3.

11 Linda Bacon and Amee Severson, "Fat Is Not the Problem—Fat Stigma
    Is," *Scientific American* Observations Blog, July 8, 2019, https://blogs
    .scientificamerican.com/observations/fat-is-not-the-problem-fat-stigma-is/.

12 Michael Hobbes, "Everything You Know about Obesity Is Wrong," Huff-
    Post, September 19, 2018, https://highline.huffingtonpost.com/articles
    /en/everything-you-know-about-obesity-is-wrong/.

13 Aubrey Gordon, *What We Don't Talk about When We Talk about Fat*
    (Boston: Beacon, 2020), 25.

14 Bacon and Severson, "Fat Is Not the Problem."

15 Jeff Yang, "Barbie's Absurd Proportions Are Hurting Mattel's Bottom
    Line," Quartz, February 11, 2014, https://qz.com/175984/barbies-absurd
    -proportions-are-hurting-mattels-bottom-line/.

16 Emma Bedford, "Barbie Sales Mattel Worldwide 2020," Statista, March
    5, 2021, www.statista.com/statistics/370361/gross-sales-of-mattel-s
    -barbie-brand/.

17 Sonya Renee Taylor, *The Body Is Not an Apology: The Power of Radical Self-
    Love* (Oakland, CA: Berrett-Koehler, 2018), 85; Bethany Biron, "Beauty Has
    Blown up to Be a \$532 Billion Industry—and Analysts Say That These 4
    Trends Will Make It Even Bigger," Business Insider, July 9, 2019, www
    .businessinsider.com/beauty-multibillion-industry-trends-future-2019-7.

18 Audre Lorde, "Age, Race, Class, and Sex: Women Redefining Differ-
    ence," in *Sister Outsider: Essays and Speeches* (1984; repr., Berkeley, CA:
    Crossing, 2015), 116.

19 Kelly Diels, "'The Perfect Woman' Is a Form of Violence against Women," October 13, 2016, https://www.kellydiels.com/perfect-woman-violence -against-women/.

20 Lorde, "Age, Race, Class, and Sex," 116.

21 Thomas Curran and Andrew P. Hill, "Perfectionism Is Increasing, and That's Not Good News," *Harvard Business Review*, January 26, 2018, https://hbr.org/2018/01/perfectionism-is-increasing-and-thats-not -good-news.

22 Tia Osborne, "Why Are the Fiverr Ads So Annoying?," Medium, June 17, 2018, https://medium.com/@tmarieos324/why-are-the-fiverr-ads -so-annoying-5c111a73b8b1.

23 Derek Thompson, "Workism Is Making Americans Miserable," *Atlantic*, August 13, 2019, www.theatlantic.com/ideas/archive/2019/02/religion -workism-making-americans-miserable/583441/.

24 Lawrence Mishel, Elise Gould, and Josh Bivens, "Wage Stagnation in Nine Charts," Economic Policy Institute, January 5, 2015, https://www .epi.org/publication/charting-wage-stagnation/; Greg Iacurci, "U.S. Is Worst among Developed Nations for Worker Benefits," CNBC, February 4, 2021, www.cnbc.com/2021/02/04/us-is-worst-among-rich -nations-for-worker-benefits.html.

25 Jia Tolentino, "The Gig Economy Celebrates Working Yourself to Death," *New Yorker*, March 22, 2017, www.newyorker.com/culture/jia-tolentino /the-gig-economy-celebrates-working-yourself-to-death.

26 Mishel, Gould, and Bivens, "Wage Stagnation in Nine Charts."

27 "From Banks and Tanks to Cooperation and Caring: A Strategic Framework for a Just Transition," Movement Generation Justice and Ecology Project, accessed September 8, 2021, https://movementgeneration.org /wp-content/uploads/2016/11/JT_booklet_Eng_printspreads.pdf, 7.

28 "From Banks and Tanks," 9.

29 Drew DeSilver, "For Most Americans, Real Wages Have Barely Budged for Decades," Pew Research Center, August 7, 2018, www.pewresearch .org/fact-tank/2018/08/07/for-most-us-workers-real-wages-have-barely -budged-for-decades/.

30 Iacurci, "Worst among Developed Nations."

31 Elise Gould and Valerie Wilson, "Black Workers Face Two of the Most Lethal Preexisting Conditions for Coronavirus—Racism and Economic Inequality," Economic Policy Institute, June 1, 2020, www.epi.org /publication/black-workers-covid/.

32 Jenny Odell, *How to Do Nothing: Resisting the Attention Economy* (New York: Melville House, 2020).

33 Talila Lewis and Dustin Gibson, "Ableism 2020: An Updated Definition," January 25, 2020, www.talilalewis.com/blog/ableism-2020-an-updated-definition.

34 Chris Costello, "How Capitalism Contributes to Ableism," The Mighty, October 29, 2017, https://themighty.com/2017/10/how-capitalism-contributes-to-ableism/.

35 Costello, "How Capitalism Contributes to Ableism."

36 Johann Hari, *Lost Connections: Why You're Depressed and How to Find Hope* (New York: Bloomsbury, 2018), 313.

37 Lynne Twist, *The Soul of Money: Reclaiming the Wealth of Our Inner Resources* (New York: W. W. Norton, 2003), 7.

38 Alexis Shotwell, *Against Purity: Living Ethically in Compromised Times* (Minneapolis: University of Minnesota Press, 2016).

39 Brené Brown, *Rising Strong: How the Ability to Reset Transforms the Way We Live, Love, Parent, and Lead* (New York: Random House, 2017), 45.

40 Brené Brown, *Daring Greatly: How the Courage to Be Vulnerable Transforms the Way We Live, Love, Parent, and Lead* (New York: Avery, 2012), 69.

41 Twist, *Soul of Money*, 209.

42 "Universal Declaration of Human Rights," United Nations, accessed September 8, 2021, www.un.org/en/about-us/universal-declaration-of-human-rights.

43 Lee Alan Dugatkin, "The Prince of Evolution: Peter Kropotkin's Adventures in Science and Politics," *Scientific American*, September 13, 2011, www.scientificamerican.com/article/the-prince-of-evolution-peter-kropotkin/.

44 Riane Eisler, *The Real Wealth of Nations* (San Francisco: Berrett-Koehler, 2007), 17.

Chapter 5

1 Jon Krakauer, *Into the Wild* (New York: Anchor Books, 1996), 189. This is a margin note that Chris McCandless wrote while reading *Doctor Zhivago*.

2 Samuel Smiles, *Self Help: With Illustrations of Character and Conduct* (Classic Reprint) (1859; repr., Ann Arbor: University of Michigan Museum of Zoology, 2012), 1.

3   Steve Chawkins, "John Vasconcellos Dies at 82; Father of California Self-Esteem Panel," *Los Angeles Times*, May 25, 2014, www.latimes.com/local/obituaries/la-me-john-vasconcellos-20140526-story.html.

4   Mark Manson, *The Subtle Art of Not Giving a F*ck: A Counterintuitive Approach to Living a Good Life* (New York: Harper, 2016).

5   John LaRosa, "$10.4 Billion Self-Improvement Market Pivots to Virtual Delivery during the Pandemic," Market Research Blog, August 2, 2021, https://blog.marketresearch.com/10.4-billion-self-improvement-market-pivots-to-virtual-delivery-during-the-pandemic.

6   "Our Philosophy," Lululemon Athletica, accessed September 13, 2021, https://shop.lululemon.com/designs/_/N-1z14oxkZ1z13xio.

7   Derek Thompson, "Workism Is Making Americans Miserable," *Atlantic*, February 24, 2019, www.theatlantic.com/ideas/archive/2019/02/religion-workism-making-americans-miserable/583441/.

8   "#Selfcare: 54,558,542 Posts," Instagram, accessed October 22, 2021, www.instagram.com/explore/tags/selfcare/.

9   Shayla Love, "The Dark Truths behind Our Obsession with Self-Care," Vice, December 11, 2018, www.vice.com/en/article/zmdwm4/the-young-and-the-uncared-for-v25n4.

10 Laurie Penny, "Life-Hacks of the Poor and Aimless," *Baffler*, July 8, 2016, https://thebaffler.com/war-of-nerves/laurie-penny-self-care.

11 "Don't Be Evil: Fred Turner on Utopias, Frontiers, and Brogrammers" (interview), *Logic*, no. 3 (December 2017), https://logicmag.io/justice/fred-turner-dont-be-evil/.

12 "Social Media Copies Gambling Methods 'to Create Psychological Cravings,'" *Guardian*, May 8, 2018, www.theguardian.com/technology/2018/may/08/social-media-copies-gambling-methods-to-create-psychological-cravings.

13 Elia Abi-Jaoude, Karline Treurnicht Naylor, and Antonio Pignatiello, "Smartphones, Social Media Use and Youth Mental Health," *Canadian Medical Association Journal* 192, no. 6 (February 2020): E136–41, https://doi.org/10.1503/cmaj.190434.

14 Jean M. Twenge and W. Keith Campbell, "The Narcissism Epidemic: Living in the Age of Entitlement," in *The Narcissism Epidemic: Living in the Age of Entitlement* (New York: Atria, 2009), 2.

15 Brad J. Bushman et al., "Looking Again, and Harder, for a Link between Low Self-Esteem and Aggression," *Journal of Personality* 77, no. 2 (2009): 427–46, https://doi.org/10.1111/j.1467-6494.2008.00553.x.

16 Ronald Butt, "Mrs Thatcher: The First Two Years," *Sunday Times*, May 3, 1981, www.margaretthatcher.org/document/104475.

17 Will Storr, *Selfie: How We Became So Self-Obsessed and What It's Doing to Us* (London: Picador, 2018), 182.

18 Storr, *Selfie*, 263.

19 Pat MacDonald, "Narcissism in the Modern World," *Psychodynamic Practice* 20, no. 2 (2014): 144–53, https://doi.org/10.1080/14753634.2014.894225.

20 Shainna Ali, "What You Need to Know about the Loneliness Epidemic," *Psychology Today*, July 12, 2018, www.psychologytoday.com/us/blog/modern-mentality/201807/what-you-need-know-about-the-loneliness-epidemic.

21 "Cigna 2018 U.S. Loneliness Index," Cigna, accessed September 13, 2021, www.cigna.com/assets/docs/newsroom/loneliness-survey-2018-fact-sheet.pdf.

22 Raheel Mushtaq et al., "Relationship between Loneliness, Psychiatric Disorders and Physical Health? A Review on the Psychological Aspects of Loneliness," *Journal of Clinical and Diagnostic Research* 8, no. 9 (September 2014): WE01–04, https://dx.doi.org/10.7860%2FJCDR%2F2014%2F10077.4828.

23 Angus Chen, "Loneliness May Warp Our Genes, and Our Immune Systems," NPR, November 29, 2015, www.npr.org/sections/health-shots/2015/11/29/457255876/loneliness-may-warp-our-genes-and-our-immune-systems.

24 "The 'Loneliness Epidemic,'" US Health Resources and Services Administration (US Department of Health and Human Services), January 10, 2019, www.hrsa.gov/enews/past-issues/2019/january-17/loneliness-epidemic.

25 "Drug Overdose Deaths," Centers for Disease Control and Prevention, March 3, 2021, www.cdc.gov/drugoverdose/deaths/index.html.

26 Nadia Kounang, "US Heroin Deaths Jump 533% since 2002, Report Says," CNN, September 8, 2017, www.cnn.com/2017/09/08/health/heroin-deaths-samhsa-report/index.html.

27 Rachel Wurzman, "How Isolation Fuels Opioid Addiction," video, TEDx Talk, October 2017, www.ted.com/talks/rachel_wurzman_how_isolation_fuels_opioid_addiction.

28 Robert D. Putnam, *Bowling Alone: Revised and Updated: The Collapse and Revival of American Community* (New York: Simon & Schuster, 2020).

29 Matt Davis, "Maslow's Forgotten Pinnacle: Self-Transcendence," Big Think, September 12, 2019, https://bigthink.com/personal-growth/maslow-self-transcendence.

30 Abraham H. Maslow, *The Farther Reaches of Human Nature* (New York: Viking, 1971), 4.

31 Teju Ravilochan with Vidya Ravilochan and Colette Kessler, "Could the Blackfoot Wisdom That Inspired Maslow Guide Us Now?," GatherFor, April 4, 2021, https://gatherfor.medium.com/maslow-got-it-wrong-ae45d6217a8c.

32 Parker J. Palmer, *A Hidden Wholeness: The Journey Toward an Undivided Life* (San Francisco: Jossey-Bass, 2004), 39.

33 Thich Nhat Hanh, "The Insight of Interbeing," Garrison Institute, August 2, 2017, www.garrisoninstitute.org/blog/insight-of-interbeing/.

34 Brené Brown, "Dare to Lead," accessed September 26, 2021, https://daretolead.brenebrown.com/.

35 Jack Kornfield, *Buddha's Little Instruction Book* (New York: Bantam Books, 1994), 28.

36 Audre Lorde, *A Burst of Light and Other Essays* (Mineola, NY: Ixia, 2017), 130.

37 Candace Reels (@femalecollective), Instagram, June 3, 2020, www.instagram.com/p/CA_Nx45gPn-/.

38 Grace Lee Boggs, *Living for Change: An Autobiography* (Minneapolis: University of Minnesota Press, 2016), 153.

39 adrienne maree brown, *We Will Not Cancel Us: And Other Dreams of Transformative Justice* (Chico, CA: AK Press, 2021).

40 adrienne maree brown, *Emergent Strategy: Shaping Change, Changing Worlds* (Chico, CA: AK Press, 2017), 218.

41 Martin Luther King Jr., "A Christmas Sermon on Peace, 1967," video, December 3, 2014, https://youtu.be/1jeyIAH3bUI.

42 john a. powell and Stephen Menendian, "The Problem of Othering: Towards Inclusiveness and Belonging," Othering and Belonging Institute, August 29, 2018, https://otheringandbelonging.org/the-problem-of-othering/.

43 john a. powell, *Racing to Justice: Transforming Our Conceptions of Self and Other to Build an Inclusive Society* (Bloomington: Indiana University Press, 2015), 228.

44 Peter Block, *Community: The Structure of Belonging* (San Francisco: Berrett-Koehler, 2008), 137–39.

Chapter 6

1 Layla Saad, *Me and White Supremacy: Combat Racism, Change the World, and Become a Good Ancestor* (Naperville, IL: Sourcebooks, 2020), 35.

2 Teju Cole, "The White-Savior Industrial Complex," *Atlantic*, March 21, 2012, www.theatlantic.com/international/archive/2012/03/the-white-savior-industrial-complex/254843/.

3 Anand Giridharadas, *Winners Take All: The Elite Charade of Changing the World* (New York: Vintage, 2018), 11.

4 Dorian O. Burton and Brian C. B. Barnes, "Shifting Philanthropy from Charity to Justice," *Stanford Social Innovation Review*, January 3, 2017, https://ssir.org/articles/entry/shifting_philanthropy_from_charity_to_justice.

5 Martin Luther King Jr., *Strength to Love* (1963; repr., Minneapolis, MN: Fortress, 2010), 25.

6 Oscar Wilde, *The Soul of Man under Socialism* (1891; repr., Whithorn, Scotland: Anodos Books, 2017), 1.

7 "Whole Foods CEO John Mackey Calling Obamacare Fascist Is Tip of the Iceberg," *Guardian*, January 18, 2013, www.theguardian.com/business/us-news-blog/2013/jan/18/whole-foods-john-mackey-fascist.

8 Ben Gilbert, "How Billionaires like Jeff Bezos and Elon Musk Avoid Paying Federal Income Tax While Increasing Their Net Worth by Billions," Business Insider, June 13, 2021, www.businessinsider.com/how-billionaires-avoid-paying-federal-income-tax-2021-6.

9 Audre Lorde, "The Master's Tools Will Never Dismantle the Master's House," in *Sister Outsider: Essays and Speeches* (1984; repr., Berkeley, CA: Crossing, 2007), 112.

10 Denise Lu, Jon Huang, Ashwin Seshagiri, Haeyoun Park, and Troy Griggs, "Faces of Power: 80% Are White, Even as U.S. Becomes More Diverse," *New York Times*, September 9, 2020, www.nytimes.com/interactive/2020/09/09/us/powerful-people-race-us.html.

11 James Baldwin, "On Being White . . . and Other Lies," Anti-Racism Digital Library, accessed September 12, 2021, https://sacred.omeka.net/items/show/238. (Originally published in *Essence*, April 1984, 90–92)

12 Isabel Wilkerson, "America's Enduring Caste System," *New York Times*, July 1, 2020, www.nytimes.com/2020/07/01/magazine/isabel-wilkerson-caste.html.

13 Wilkerson, "America's Enduring Caste System."

14 Robin D. G. Kelley, "What Did Cedric Robinson Mean by Racial Capitalism?," *Boston Review*, January 12, 2017, https://bostonreview.net/race/robin-d-g-kelley-what-did-cedric-robinson-mean-racial-capitalism.

15 Ibram X. Kendi, *How to Be an Antiracist* (New York: One World, 2019), 42.

16 Michelle Alexander, *The New Jim Crow: Mass Incarceration in the Age of Colorblindness*, 10th anniv. ed. (2010; repr., New York: New Press, 2020).

17 Wilkerson, *Caste*, 141.

18 Elizabeth Currid-Halkett, *The Sum of Small Things: A Theory of the Aspirational Class* (Princeton, NJ: Princeton University Press, 2017).

19 Brené Brown and Sonya Renee Taylor, "Brené with Sonya Renee Taylor on 'The Body Is Not an Apology,'" September 16, 2020, *Unlocking Us* podcast, https://brenebrown.com/podcast/brene-with-sonya-renee-taylor-on-the-body-is-not-an-apology/.

20 Mike Baker et al., "Three Words. 70 Cases. The Tragic History of 'I Can't Breathe,'" *New York Times*, June 29, 2020, www.nytimes.com/interactive/2020/06/28/us/i-cant-breathe-police-arrest.html.

21 Michelle C. Johnson, *Skill in Action: Radicalizing Your Yoga Practice to Create a Just World* (Boulder, CO: Shambhala, 2020), 14.

22 "Risk for COVID-19 Infection, Hospitalization, and Death by Race/Ethnicity," Centers for Disease Control and Prevention, September 9, 2021, www.cdc.gov/coronavirus/2019-ncov/covid-data/investigations-discovery/hospitalization-death-by-race-ethnicity.html.

23 Karissa Knapp, "Police: Sixth-Leading Cause of Death for Young Black Men," Institute for Social Research (University of Michigan), June 1, 2020, https://isr.umich.edu/news-events/news-releases/police-sixth-leading-cause-of-death-for-young-black-men-2/.

24 Dorothy Roberts, "Abolishing Policing Also Means Abolishing Family Regulation," The Imprint, June 16, 2020, https://imprintnews.org/child-welfare-2/abolishing-policing-also-means-abolishing-family-regulation/44480.

25 Tom Loveless, "2017 Brown Center Report on American Education: Race and School Suspensions," Brookings, March 22, 2017, www.brookings.edu/research/2017-brown-center-report-part-iii-race-and-school-suspensions/.

26 Tema Okun, "Characteristics," White Supremacy Culture, accessed September 12, 2021, www.whitesupremacyculture.info/characteristics.html.

27 Martin Luther King Jr., "Letter from a Birmingham Jail," African Studies Center, University of Pennsylvania, accessed September 12, 2021, www.africa.upenn.edu/Articles_Gen/Letter_Birmingham.html.

28 Stephanie E. Jones-Rogers, *They Were Her Property: White Women as Slave Owners in the American South* (New Haven, CT: Yale University Press, 2019), xvii.

29 Sarah Lamble, "Practising Everyday Abolition," Abolitionist Futures, August 19, 2020, https://abolitionistfutures.com/latest-news/practising-everyday-abolition.

30 Rev. angel Kyodo williams, Lama Rod Owens, and Jasmine Syedullah, *Radical Dharma: Talking Race, Love, and Liberation* (Berkeley, CA: North Atlantic Books, 2016), xxvi.

31 williams, Owens, and Syedullah, *Radical Dharma*, 182.

32 Kyle "Guante" Tran Myhre, "'White Supremacy Is Not a Shark; It Is the Water," Not a Lot of Reasons to Sing, but Enough, November 22, 2020, https://guante.info/2020/11/22/nottheshark/#more-3860.

33 Eula Biss, "White Debt," *New York Times*, December 6, 2015, www.nytimes.com/2015/12/06/magazine/white-debt.html.

34 Rebecca Nagle, "Invisibility Is the Modern Form of Racism Against Native Americans," *Teen Vogue*, October 23, 2018, www.teenvogue.com/story/racism-against-native-americans.

35 Bob Burnett, "If You're Black, Get Back," HuffPost, May 25, 2011, www.huffpost.com/entry/if-youre-black-get-back_b_21426.

36 Matthew Lee, "Coronavirus Fears Show How 'Model Minority' Asian Americans Become the 'Yellow Peril,'" NBC News, March 12, 2020, www.nbcnews.com/think/opinion/coronavirus-fears-show-how-model-minority-asian-americans-become-yellow-ncna1151671.

37 Louise A Cainkar, *Homeland Insecurity: The Arab American and Muslim American Experience after 9/11* (New York, NY: Russell Sage Foundation, 2009).

38 Brennan Hoban, "Do Immigrants 'Steal' Jobs from American Workers?," Brookings, July 19, 2018, www.brookings.edu/blog/brookings-now/2017/08/24/do-immigrants-steal-jobs-from-american-workers/.

39 Dave Davies, "'Sum of Us' Examines the Hidden Cost of Racism—for Everyone," NPR, February 17, 2021, www.npr.org/2021/02/17/968638759/sum-of-us-examines-the-hidden-cost-of-racism-for-everyone.

40 *Mental Health: Culture, Race, and Ethnicity: A Supplement to Mental Health: A Report of the Surgeon General*, US Department of Health and Human Services, 2001, https://www.ncbi.nlm.nih.gov/books/NBK44246/.

41 Atul Gawande, "Why Americans Are Dying from Despair," *New Yorker*, March 16, 2020, www.newyorker.com/magazine/2020/03/23/why-americans-are-dying-from-despair.

42 James Baldwin, *No Name in the Street* (1972; repr., New York: Vintage International, 2007), 54.

43 John Schmitt and Janelle Jones, "Slow Progress for Fast-Food Workers," Center for Economic and Policy Research, August 2013, https://cepr.net/documents/publications/fast-food-workers-2013-08.pdf.

44 "Step Four," Working the Steps, accessed September 12, 2021, www.therecoverygroup.org/wts/2002/2002-04q4.html.

45 Sonya Renee Taylor, Instagram, March 9, 2019, www.instagram.com/p/BuzYggqBkIl/.

46 Brené Brown and Austin Channing Brown, "Brené with Austin Channing Brown on I'm Still Here: Black Dignity in a World Made for Whiteness" June 10, 2020, *Unlocking Us* podcast, https://brenebrown.com/podcast/brene-with-austin-channing-brown-on-im-still-here-black-dignity-in-a-world-made-for-whiteness/.

47 Mia Mingus, "The Four Parts of Accountability: How to Give a Genuine Apology Part 1," Leaving Evidence, December 18, 2019, https://leavingevidence.wordpress.com/2019/12/18/how-to-give-a-good-apology-part-1-the-four-parts-of-accountability/.

48 Walidah Imarisha et al., "The Fictions and Futures of Transformative Justice," New Inquiry, April 20, 2017, https://thenewinquiry.com/the-fictions-and-futures-of-transformative-justice/.

49 Ruth Wilson Gilmore, "Making Abolition Geography in California's Central Valley," interview by Léopold Lambert, *Funambulist*, no. 21, December 20, 2018, https://thefunambulist.net/magazine/21-space-activism/interview-making-abolition-geography-california-central-valley-ruth-wilson-gilmore.

50 Sarah Lamble, "Practising Everyday Abolition," Abolitionist Futures, August 19, 2020, https://abolitionistfutures.com/latest-news/practising-everyday-abolition.

51 Darnell L. Moore, "Foreword: Love Is a Reckoning," in *Love WITH Accountability: Digging Up the Roots of Child Sexual Abuse*, ed. Aishah Shahidah Simmons (Chico, CA: AK Press, 2020).

Chapter 7

1 Stephanie Savell, Catherine Lutz, and Neta Crawford, "Costs of the 20-Year War on Terror: $8 Trillion and 900,000 Deaths," Costs of War Project (Brown University), September 1, 2021, www.brown.edu /news/2021-09-01/costsofwar.

2 Martin Gilens and Benjamin I. Page, "Testing Theories of American Politics: Elites, Interest Groups, and Average Citizens," *Perspectives on Politics* 12, no. 3 (2014): 564–81, https://doi.org/10.1017/S1537592714001595.

3 Eli Yokley, "Voters Are Nearly United in Support for Expanded Background Checks," Morning Consult, March 10, 2021, https://morningconsult.com /2021/03/10/house-gun-legislation-background-checks-polling/; Gaby Galvin, "About 7 in 10 Voters Favor a Public Health Insurance Option. Medicare for All Remains Polarizing," Morning Consult, March 23, 2021, https://morningconsult.com/2021/03/24/medicare-for-all-public-option -polling/; Howard Schneider and Chris Kahn, "Majority of Americans Favor Wealth Tax on Very Rich: Reuters/Ipsos Poll," Reuters, January 10, 2020, https://www.reuters.com/article/us-usa-election-inequality-poll /majority-of-americans-favor-wealth-tax-on-very-rich-reuters-ipsos -poll-idUSKBN1Z9141; Alec Tyson and Brian Kennedy, "Two-Thirds of Americans Think Government Should Do More on Climate," Pew Research Center, July 12, 2021, www.pewresearch.org/science/2020/06/23 /two-thirds-of-americans-think-government-should-do-more-on-climate/.

4 Jeffrey M. Jones, "Quarterly Gap in Party Affiliation Largest since 2012," Gallup, August 13, 2021, https://news.gallup.com/poll/343976/quarterly -gap-party-affiliation-largest-2012.aspx.

5 Robert D. Putnam, *Bowling Alone: Revised and Updated: The Collapse and Revival of American Community* (New York: Simon & Schuster, 2020).

6 Carol Hanisch, "The Personal Is Political: The Women's Liberation Movement Classic with a New Explanatory Introduction," accessed September 12, 2021, www.carolhanisch.org/CHwritings/PIP.html.

7 "H. R. 40, Naturalization Bill, March 4, 1790," US Capitol Visitor Center, accessed September 13, 2021, www.visitthecapitol.gov/exhibitions /artifact/h-r-40-naturalization-bill-march-4-1790.

8 Nicole Prchal Svajlenka, "Protecting Undocumented Workers on the Pandemic's Front Lines," Center for American Progress, December 2, 2020, www.americanprogress.org/issues/immigration/reports/2020/12/02/493307 /protecting-undocumented-workers-pandemics-front-lines/.

9   Karolina Chorvath and Jose Antonio Vargas, "After Pittsburgh, Jose Antonio Vargas Asks, 'Who Is an American?,'" *The World*, October 30, 2018, https://www.pri.org/stories/2018-10-30/jose-antonio-vargas-who-american.

10 "Immigration Act of 1924 (Johnson-Reed Act)," Immigration History, February 1, 2020, https://immigrationhistory.org/item/1924-immigration-act-johnson-reed-act/.

11 "December 6, 1923: First Annual Message," Miller Center, February 23, 2017, https://millercenter.org/the-presidency/presidential-speeches/december-6-1923-first-annual-message.

12 Ibram X. Kendi, "The Day *Shithole* Entered the Presidential Lexicon," *Atlantic*, January 27, 2020), www.theatlantic.com/politics/archive/2019/01/shithole-countries/580054/.

13 Dale C. Tatum, "How a Failed 17th Century Rebellion Can Help Explain Donald Trump's Election Victory," LSE Phelan US Centre, September 18, 2017, https://blogs.lse.ac.uk/usappblog/2017/09/13/how-a-failed-17th-century-rebellion-can-help-explain-donald-trumps-election-victory/.

14 Heather McGhee, *The Sum of Us: What Racism Costs Everyone and How We Can Prosper Together* (New York: One World, 2021), 9.

15 Ian Haney López, *Dog Whistle Politics: How Coded Racial Appeals Have Reinvented Racism and Wrecked the Middle Class* (New York: Oxford University Press, 2014).

16 William H. Frey, "The US Will Become 'Minority White' in 2045, Census Projects," Brookings, September 10, 2018, www.brookings.edu/blog/the-avenue/2018/03/14/the-us-will-become-minority-white-in-2045-census-projects/.

17 Paul Rosenberg, "A Unifying 'Race-Class Narrative': Blueprint for Progressive Victory?," Salon, June 10, 2018, www.salon.com/2018/06/10/a-unifying-race-class-narrative-blueprint-for-progressive-victory/.

18 Umair Haque, "The Birth of Predatory Capitalism: How the Free World Took Four Giant Leaps to Self-Destruction," Eudaimonia and Co., March 3, 2019, https://eand.co/the-birth-of-predatory-capitalism-6d443eda03.

19 Patrick Berry et al., "Voting Laws Roundup: May 2021," Brennan Center for Justice, May 28, 2021, www.brennancenter.org/our-work/research-reports/voting-laws-roundup-may-2021.

20 Lindsey Graham (@LindseyGrahamSC), "I'm disappointed to hear the House is proceeding with a second impeachment given there are only nine days left in a Trump presidency...," Twitter, January 11, 2021, https://twitter.com/lindseygrahamsc/status/1348732263958257668.

21 Democracy for America (@DFAaction), "@DFAaction CEO @Ysimpson-power on the Road Ahead…," Twitter, November 7, 2020, https://twitter.com/DFAaction/status/1325153722985402375.

22 "Alicia Garza on Identity Politics and 2020 US Presidential Election," *Who Belongs?* podcast, ep. 17, December 2, 2019, Othering and Belonging Institute, https://belonging.berkeley.edu/whobelongs/identitypolitics.

23 Laverne Cox, "Trans People Have a Right to Exist in Public Space with Equal Access," Instagram, February 23, 2017, www.instagram.com/p/BQ23u6FAoOU/.

24 "The Combahee River Collective Statement," Combahee River Collective, accessed September 12, 2021, https://combaheerivercollective.weebly.com/the-combahee-river-collective-statement.html.

25 Katy Steinmetz, "Kimberlé Crenshaw on What Intersectionality Means Today," *Time*, February 20, 2020, https://time.com/5786710/kimberle-crenshaw-intersectionality/.

26 Alicia Garza, "Identity Politics: Friend or Foe?," Othering and Belonging Institute, September 24, 2019, https://belonging.berkeley.edu/identity-politics-friend-or-foe.

27 Yanna Krupnikov and John Barry Ryan, "The Real Divide in America Is between Political Junkies and Everyone Else," *New York Times*, October 20, 2020, https://www.nytimes.com/2020/10/20/opinion/polarization-politics-americans.html.

28 "Elie Wiesel," Oxford Reference, accessed September 12, 2021, https://www.oxfordreference.com/view/10.1093/acref/9780191826719.001.0001/q-oro-ed4-00011516.

29 Rana Sodhi and Harjit Sodhi, "Remembering Balbir Singh Sodhi, Sikh Man Killed in Post-9/11 Hate Crime," StoryCorps, September 13, 2018, https://storycorps.org/stories/remembering-balbir-singh-sodhi-sikh-man-killed-in-post-911-hate-crime/.

30 Jane Mulcahy, "The Human Condition: We Are All on a Quest for Safety," PACEsConnection, March 31, 2020, www.pacesconnection.com/blog/the-human-condition-we-are-all-on-a-quest-for-safety.

31 Mark Gonzales, in discussion with the author, August 5, 2020.

32 john a. powell, "Bridging or Breaking? The Stories We Tell Will Create the Future We Inhabit," *Nonprofit Quarterly*, February 15, 2021, https://nonprofitquarterly.org/bridging-or-breaking-the-stories-we-tell-will-create-the-future-we-inhabit/.

33 Peter Block, *Community: The Structure of Belonging* (San Francisco: Berrett-Koehler, 2008), 63.

34 Rebecca Solnit, *A Paradise Built in Hell: The Extraordinary Communities That Arise in Disaster* (New York: Penguin Books, 2010).

35 Rebecca Solnit, *Hope in the Dark: Untold Histories, Wild Possibilities* (Chicago: Haymarket Books, 2016), 24.

36 Solnit, *Paradise Built in Hell*, 7.

37 Xan West, Kazu Haga, LCF8M, and Carinne Luck, "Can Our Movements Be the Healing?," *CTZN* podcast, January 8, 2021, CTZNWELL, www .ctznwell.org/ctznpodcast/can-our-movements-be-healing-xan-west-kazu -haga-lcf8m-carinne-luck.

38 bell hooks, *Writing Beyond Race: Living Theory and Practice* (New York: Routledge, 2013), 4.

39 "Combahee River Collective Statement," Combahee River Collective.

40 Grace Lee Boggs, "Visionary Organizing and the MLK Memorial," Boggs Blog (James and Grace Lee Boggs Center to Nurture Community Leadership), September 3, 2011, https://conversationsthatyouwillneverfinish .wordpress.com/2011/09/05/visionary-organizing-and-the-mlk-memorial -by-grace-lee-boggs/.

41 Martin Luther King Jr., "Beyond Vietnam" (speech, Riverside Church, New York City, April 4, 1967), African-American Involvement in the Vietnam War, www.aavw.org/special_features/speeches_speech_king01.html.

42 Solnit, *Hope in the Dark*, 4.

43 "Media Toolkit," #WeGovern, accessed October 21, 2021, https:// we-govern.org/#media-toolkit.

Chapter 8

1 adrienne maree brown, *Emergent Strategy: Shaping Change, Changing Worlds* (AK Press, 2017), 20.

2 Taj James, "Follow the Ones Who Know the Way...," Facebook, June 19, 2021, www.facebook.com/taj.james/posts/10158639535497606.

3 Arundhati Roy, *Azadi: Freedom. Fascism. Fiction.* (Chicago: Haymarket Books, 2020), 213–14, Kindle.

Epilogue

1 *Oxford Lexico US Dictionary*, s.v. "emergence," accessed October 21, 2021, www.lexico.com/en/definition/emergence.

INDEX

ABOUT THE AUTHOR

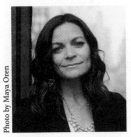

KERRI KELLY is the founder of CTZNWELL, a movement that is democratizing well-being for all. A descendant of generations of firemen and first responders, Kerri has dedicated her life to kicking down doors and fighting for justice. She's been teaching yoga for more than twenty years and is known for making waves in the wellness industry by challenging norms, disrupting systems, and mobilizing people to act.

A community organizer and wellness activist, Kerri is recognized across communities for her inspired work to bridge transformational practice with social justice. She's been instrumental in translating the practices of well-being into social and political action, working in collaboration with community organizers, spiritual leaders, and policy makers to transform our systems from the inside out. Her leadership has inspired a movement that is actively organizing around issues of racial and economic justice, healthcare as a human right, civic engagement, and more.

Kerri is a powerful facilitator, TED speaker, and host of the prominent podcast *CTZN*. You can learn more about her work at https://kerrikelly.co and https://ctznwell.org.

About North Atlantic Books

North Atlantic Books (NAB) is a 501(c)(3) nonprofit publisher committed to a bold exploration of the relationships between mind, body, spirit, culture, and nature. Founded in 1974, NAB aims to nurture a holistic view of the arts, sciences, humanities, and healing. To make a donation or to learn more about our books, authors, events, and newsletter, please visit www.northatlanticbooks.com.